Nursing Leadership During Crisis

Insights Guiding Leaders From the Covid-19 Pandemic

Carolyn Miller Reilly
Barbara Kaplan
Tim Porter-O'Grady

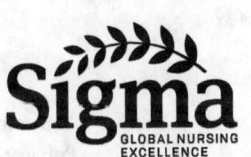

Copyright © 2023 by Sigma Theta Tau International Honor Society of Nursing

All rights reserved. This book is protected by copyright. No part of it may be reproduced, stored in a retrieval system, or transmitted in any form or by any means, electronic, mechanical, photocopying, recording, or otherwise, without written permission from the publisher. Any trademarks, service marks, design rights, or similar rights that are mentioned, used, or cited in this book are the property of their respective owners. Their use here does not imply that you may use them for a similar or any other purpose.

This book is not intended to be a substitute for the medical advice of a licensed medical professional. The author and publisher have made every effort to ensure the accuracy of the information contained within at the time of its publication and shall have no liability or responsibility to any person or entity regarding any loss or damage incurred, or alleged to have incurred, directly or indirectly, by the information contained in this book. The author and publisher make no warranties, express or implied, with respect to its content, and no warranties may be created or extended by sales representatives or written sales materials. The author and publisher have no responsibility for the consistency or accuracy of URLs and content of third-party websites referenced in this book.

Sigma Theta Tau International Honor Society of Nursing (Sigma) is a nonprofit organization whose mission is developing nurse leaders anywhere to improve healthcare everywhere. Founded in 1922, Sigma has more than 135,000 active members in over 100 countries and territories. Members include practicing nurses, instructors, researchers, policymakers, entrepreneurs, and others. Sigma's more than 540 chapters are located at more than 700 institutions of higher education throughout Armenia, Australia, Botswana, Brazil, Canada, Colombia, Croatia, England, Eswatini, Ghana, Hong Kong, Ireland, Israel, Italy, Jamaica, Japan, Jordan, Kenya, Lebanon, Malawi, Mexico, the Netherlands, Nigeria, Pakistan, Philippines, Portugal, Puerto Rico, Scotland, Singapore, South Africa, South Korea, Sweden, Taiwan, Tanzania, Thailand, the United States, and Wales. Learn more at www.sigmanursing.org.

Sigma Theta Tau International
550 West North Street
Indianapolis, IN, USA 46202

To request a review copy for course adoption, order additional books, buy in bulk, or purchase for corporate use, contact Sigma Marketplace at 888.654.4968 (US/Canada toll-free), +1.317.687.2256 (International), or solutions@sigmamarketplace.org.

To request author information, or for speaker or other media requests, contact Sigma Marketing at 888.634.7575 (US/Canada toll-free) or +1.317.634.8171 (International).

ISBN:	9781646480425
EPUB ISBN:	9781646480432
PDF ISBN:	9781646480449

First Printing, 2023

Publisher: Dustin Sullivan
Acquisitions Editor: Emily Hatch
Development Editor: Meaghan O'Keeffe
Cover Designer: Rebecca Batchelor
Interior Design/Page Layout: Rebecca Batchelor
Indexer: Larry Sweazy

Managing Editor: Carla Hall
Publications Specialist: Todd Lothery
Project Editor: Meaghan O'Keeffe
Copy Editor: Erin Geile
Proofreader: Todd Lothery

Library of Congress Control Number: 2022948642

DEDICATION

This book is dedicated to all the great nursing leaders and our colleagues who informed the content of this book and inspired us over the years. From watching, listening, and walking beside you, we have developed our own ability to lead, create, adapt, collaborate, and cope.

To our loved ones and families, your patience and encouragement have never failed. Your love and dedication have allowed us to bloom. Thank you for your tender care and keeping the world moving when we struggled to see past the next deadline or find a matching shoe.

Carolyn, Barbara, and Tim

PRAISE FOR *NURSING LEADERSHIP DURING CRISIS*

"*Nursing Leadership During Crisis* provides powerful insight into the new leadership necessary for our current healthcare environment. Informed from the recent pandemic, the authors stress leading differently through influence and innovation with an emphasis on self-care and mindfulness for the leader who must care for self in order to care for and lead others. It is a must read for developing and mentoring nursing leaders."

–Kathleen M. White, PhD, RN, NEA-BC, FAAN
Professor Emeritus, Johns Hopkins School of Nursing
Chairperson, Johns Hopkins Howard County General Hospital Board of Trustees
Adjunct Faculty, Johns Hopkins School of Education
Visiting Professor, American University of Armenia

"*Nursing Leadership During Crisis* provides a clear call to action for all nurse leaders inevitably navigating the confluence of the Covid-19 pandemic and a wide range of profound societal shifts. Through a series of compelling narratives, the authors reveal the historic opportunity at hand to lead with joy and purpose through human connectedness and relationships as a path to intentionally transforming the nursing profession's impact from most trusted to most influential."

–Laura J. Wood, DNP, RN, NEA-BC, FAAN
EVP, Patient Care Operations & System Chief Nursing Officer,
Sporing Carpenter Chair for Nursing
Boston Children's Hospital

"The importance of leadership in nursing cannot be overstated. Situating leadership in today's context is the unique contribution of this book. The pandemic affected clinical practice, higher education, the workplace, and our overall society in unprecedented ways, including the economic shutdown. The shutting down of our society made racial injustice visible. The crises resulting from these challenges demand a new skill set and profile for leaders that go beyond the past personas. This book provides a road map and mechanism to develop the socially responsive leaders needed as we move to a preferred future."

–Angela Frederick Amar, PhD, RN, ANEF, FAAN
Dean and Professor
University of Nevada, Las Vegas School of Nursing

"This book will be used for generations by nurse leaders and others due to its practical and theoretical information. The authors hit on all the critical topics needed to manage a crisis and provide tools, strategies, and stories to help the reader internalize the information. I highly recommend this book for lessons on everyday leadership, as well as crisis leadership."

–Linda Wick, MSN, APRN, CHFN
Associate Chief Nurse Executive, M Health Fairview Health System
Co-chair, COVID incident command for University of Minnesota

"This book cannot be published at a better time. As we move from pandemic to endemic, readiness is key, as there will be other crises in healthcare. The authors are seasoned experts who have weaved wisdom from many disciplines into content vitally applicable for emerging leaders in today's healthcare milieus. The cutting-edge content and chapter exercises operationalize theoretical tenets to practice. Kudos to the authors for this seminal, much-needed work!"

–Lola A. Coke, PhD, ACNS-BC, FAHA, FPCNA, FANP, FAAN
Acting Dean, Kirkhof College of Nursing
Grand Valley State University

ACKNOWLEDGMENTS

Foremost, this work could not have been completed without our 2020 Accelerated Bachelor of Nursing Leadership Scholars who assisted with most phases of this qualitative research by developing questions, completing the interviews with their mentors, transcribing the recordings, and then completing initial thematic analyses. We are so thankful and proud of each as they complete their first year of practice in these unprecedented times, entering into the profession of nursing in spring 2021:

Amanda Baeten, BSN, RN
Duke University Health System, Durham, NC

Claire Duerson, BSN, RN
Southwest Medical Associates Surgery Center, Henderson, NV

Michelle Hill, BSN, RN
OhioHealth, Columbus, OH

Hannah Latham, BSN, RN
Children's Healthcare of Atlanta, Atlanta, GA

Nichole Edge Lopez, BSN, RN
Johnson City Medical Center, Ballad Health, Johnson City, TN

Tegan McEntire, BS, BSN, RN, CBC
Children's Healthcare of Atlanta, Atlanta, GA

Stephanie Daisy Nagel, BSN, RN
Duke University Hospital, Durham, NC
Case Manager, Liberty Hospice Care, Sanford NC

Vani C. Nimbal, MPH, BSN, RN
El Camino Hospital, Mountain View, CA
Epidemiologist, Applied Research Community Health Epidemiology & Surveillance (ARCHES) Branch, San Francisco Department of Public Health, San Francisco, CA

Dara Suchke, BSN, RN
Emory University Hospital Midtown, Atlanta, GA

Laura Werbaneth, BSN, RN
Grady Health System, Atlanta, GA

SPECIAL ACKNOWLEDGMENT

In December of 2019, when Covid-19 was just being recognized in Asia, 19 students in a second-degree, accelerated BSN program (ABSN) were completing their first semester at the Nell Hodgson Woodruff School of Nursing at Emory University, while vying for one of the 10 Leadership Scholars Program (LSP) openings. This honor's program promised to provide a challenging and enriching academic experience for highly motivated and engaged students desiring to become clinical leaders. Our goal was to pair students with mentors who modeled leadership daily in advocacy, policy, quality, and safety initiatives. The plan was for these LSP students to shadow the mentors over the course of 10 months, build a dynamic network through cohort and mentoring relationships, and explore nursing as an integral and leading component of healthcare delivery, culminating in a leadership project that benefited the nursing mentor's unit or facility (e.g., systems quality improvement project, policy analysis, transformative teaching, or health promotion/disease prevention project).

In January 2020, the 10 selected Leadership Scholars began to meet for weekly seminars with the faculty of this program and ultimately the editors of this book. As leaders in varied aspects of nursing practice, research, education, and service, we had coalesced as a faculty team and partnered with many of our nurse leader colleagues across the city over the past few years to mentor the next generation of nurse leaders in this program. We had just finished matching our students with their mentors over spring break (mid-March 2020) when Covid forced us to take another week to regroup and move to remote teaching, as every nurse leader was now stretched beyond reason and could not actually meet with any of their students. As we shifted from expecting this to just be a short-term situation to then something that would take months to resolve (who knew years were on the horizon?), we began to hear anecdotal stories from these nurse leaders about how leadership during the midst of this crisis was unlike anything they had ever faced—how they needed to lead differently, how there was too much information or not enough, how opinions were heard and not heard, how staff pulled together and how others quit, how they were scared for their staff and grateful to the pots-and-pans chorus by neighbors at shift change, how there were not enough supplies, and how they were having to make tough decisions for patient lives, utilization of resources, and ending family visitation.

All of our LSP students graduated in December of 2020; all passed NCLEX and secured professional nursing positions working in diverse settings, from pediatrics to ambulatory to acute care. Several have continued to stay in touch with this project, and a few have co-authored the chapters you'll read. Each had come into our program with hopes of working with one population or another, and we secured mentors complementary to their backgrounds and desired populations, placing these students with a fantastic depth and breadth of roles at the very beginning of their LSP program. Little did we know how fortunate and influential this representation from diverse areas of nursing leadership would be to shaping this book. Our mentors were from every possible level of nursing leadership, working with a multitude of populations and facing a myriad of challenges during the epidemic. We are grateful to both these mentors and the students listed who gave of themselves to develop this book in the midst of crisis leadership.

ABOUT THE AUTHORS

CAROLYN MILLER REILLY, PHD, RN, CHFN, CNE, FAHA, FAAN

Dr. Carolyn Reilly has devoted more than 30 years to caring for critically ill and cardiovascular patients, primarily as a clinical nurse specialist. It is from this point of reference that she teaches anything cardiac or vaguely related to hemodynamics. Most of Reilly's clinical research centers on promoting self-care in persons suffering from or at risk for cardiovascular disease, including several studies managing self-care and symptoms in persons with heart failure and others in preventing heart disease in cancer survivors. Reilly also has a strong leadership background, serving as a program director in both clinical and academic settings and holding executive leadership appointments in various professional organizations. She has led the Leadership Scholars Program at Emory University since its inception, has previously conducted nursing workforce retention research, is well-published, has served on national writing groups, and serves with editorial boards for several cardiovascular and critical care journals. She recently moved to Berry College in Mt. Berry, Georgia, to lead the Division of Nursing. She is devoted to her children, husband, church, and community and can often be found cheering on her teenagers at sporting events, singing in the church choir, whipping up gourmet meals and drinks, or traveling to experience new cultures and learn new recipes.

BARBARA KAPLAN, MSN, RN

Barbara Kaplan is currently an Instructor at the Emory University Nell Hodgson Woodruff School of Nursing and the Co-Director of the Veteran Affairs Nursing Academic Partnership program. Over her 41-year career, Kaplan's focus has been on undergraduate teaching, inclusive of the faculty team for the Leadership Scholars Program and mentoring of student projects within this course and other clinical courses. As one of the founders of the multifaceted simulation lab at Emory University, she served as the Lab Coordinator for many years, where her expertise lies in simulation design, implementation and evaluation, lab schematics, and faculty consultation. Kaplan has led simulation workshops at the international level, training students, interprofessional teams, and healthcare practitioners. She has presented, published, and received accolades for simulation and nursing education. She loves outdoors activities, travel, knitting, and beaming over her grandchildren.

TIM PORTER-O'GRADY, DM, EDD, SCD(H), APRN, FAAN, FACCWS

Dr. Tim Porter-O'Grady has been a nurse for 50 years. He is currently Senior Partner-Health Systems for TPOG Associates LLC, an international health consulting practice in Tucson, Arizona, and a Clinical Professor at Emory University in Atlanta, Georgia. He is an advanced practice nurse, board certified in geriatrics and wound specialties, and he holds two earned doctorates, one in learning behavior and another in complex systems leadership.

Porter-O'Grady has been a Clinical Professor and Leadership Scholar at The Ohio State University College of Nursing and Professor and Innovations Scholar at Arizona State University College of Nursing and Health Innovation. He is nationally and internationally recognized as an expert/futurist in clinical health systems, nursing leadership, nursing professional governance, and health systems innovation.

He has consulted with over 300 clinical systems worldwide and has lectured at over 500 settings globally. He has authored/co-authored 26 books and over 225 journal publications and is a 10-time winner of the AJN Book of the Year Award.

Porter-O'Grady is an elected Fellow of the American Academy of Nursing and a clinical Fellow in the American College of Clinical Wound Specialists. He is immediate past Chair of the Board of the American Nurses Foundation and currently serves on the board of Catholic Community Services, a community health system for the underserved in Tucson, Arizona. He has also served on the editorial boards of five proctored healthcare journals.

Porter-O'Grady has received numerous awards including the American Organization of Nurse Leaders Lifetime Achievement Award, American Nurses Association Luther Christman Health Leadership Award, American Association of Critical-Care Nurses Healthcare Pioneer

Award, and the American Academy of Nursing President's Award. He is a 2020 inductee into the ANA Nursing Hall of Fame and a 2022 inaugural inductee into the Georgia Nurses Hall of Fame. He loves reading and hiking the many trails in the Catalina Mountains surrounding Tucson with his husband and friends.

CONTRIBUTING AUTHORS

SHERLEY BELIZAIRE, DNP, PMHNP-BC, FNP-BC
(CHAPTERS 2 AND 3)

Dr. Belizaire is the Director of the Nurse Practitioner Residency Program-Mental Health and a Psychiatric-Mental Health Nurse Practitioner at the VA Boston Healthcare System. She developed and implemented the Psychiatric-Mental Health Nurse Practitioner Residency Program in 2014. She mentors new NP residency program directors nationally. She has more than 20 years of nursing experience in mental health, substance use disorder, and primary care. She has held multiple roles in clinical and academic settings including nursing supervisor, sexual assault nurse examiner, consultant, and nursing faculty. She holds an adjunct clinical faculty position at the Boston College William F. Connell School of Nursing. Belizaire served as an expert on the standardized competency-based nurse practitioner curriculum task force. She serves on the steering and advisory committees for post-baccalaureate and post-graduate nursing residency programs. Belizaire has received awards for "Mentoring" and "Excellence in Nursing Leadership."

LISA MUIRHEAD, DNP, ANP-BC, FAANP, FAAN
(CHAPTERS 2 AND 3)

Dr. Muirhead is the Assistant Dean for Diversity, Equity, and Inclusion and Associate Professor, at Emory University, Nell Hodgson Woodruff School of Nursing. She leads the development and strategic vision of the school's effort to build a diverse community that values the importance of equity and inclusivity. She has practiced as an APRN for greater than 25 years and has an extensive background focused on advancing health equity among underrepresented populations and Veterans' healthcare. As a recognized national expert and consultant to numerous advisory boards, national groups, and public health organizations, she has contributed to national health recommendations, state nursing guidelines, and standardized competency-based nurse practitioner curriculum. She serves on national Diversity, Equity, and Inclusion work groups to help inform educational initiatives that build capacity for a diversified faculty and nursing workforce. She has been recognized for her extraordinary leadership in nursing practice, education, and policy as a Fellow of the American Association of Nurse Practitioners and a Fellow of the American Academy of Nurses.

KATHERINE PFEIFFER, DNP, PMHNP-CNS, PMHCNS-BC (CHAPTER 9)

Dr. Pfeiffer is an Assistant Professor at the Nell Hodgson Woodruff School of Nursing, Emory University, Atlanta, GA. She has worked as a psychiatric advanced practice nurse in outpatient mental health for many years, with a focus on solution-focused therapy and wellbeing strategies. Pfeiffer also teaches psychiatric mental health nursing, as well as therapeutic and behavior-change focused communication strategies. Her clinical research interests include the phenomenon of posttraumatic growth among healthcare workers secondary to workplace traumatic experiencing, and curricular strategies to facilitate posttraumatic growth for nurse entry to practice, which include studying factors such as coping, help-seeking behavior, perceived support, and resiliency among nursing students.

ANGELA RICHARD-EAGLIN, DNP, MSN, FNP-BC, CNE, FAANP (CHAPTERS 2 AND 3)

Dr. Richard-Eaglin is the Associate Dean for Equity and an Associate Clinical Professor at Yale School of Nursing. She is a board-certified family nurse practitioner and a champion for expanding diversity and inspiring cultural intelligence (CQ) and endorsing the humanitarian ethos within healthcare organizations and health professions education programs to influence translation to clinical practice. Her nursing career spans nearly 30 years, all of which has been dedicated to advancing equity among vulnerable, underrepresented, marginalized, stigmatized, and financially disadvantaged populations. As a perpetual advocate in incessant pursuit of sustainable health equity initiatives, she became a Certified Professional Cultural Intelligence I&II and Unconscious Bias

Facilitator and Coach. Because of her assiduous commitment to health justice, social justice, and organizational cultural excellence, Richard-Eaglin develops and facilitates customized CQ workshops for all departments and across disciplines of academic and healthcare institutions. The guiding principles for her unrelenting commitment to advocacy and activism are humanitarianism and egalitarianism. Richard-Eaglin is a globally recognized leader for her dedication to and support of initiatives aimed at cultivating environments that authentically embrace differences and embody inclusive excellence.

DARA SUCHKE, BSN, RN
(CHAPTER 5)

Dara Suchke was part of the Leadership Scholars Program while studying nursing at Emory University, and she graduated with her BSN in December 2020. She is currently working on a medical-surgical nursing unit in Atlanta, GA. She is a member of Sigma Theta Tau and recently won the DAISY award. Prior to nursing, Suchke worked in education and ecological horticulture.

MICHELLE WEBB, DNP, RN, BC-CHPCA
(CHAPTERS 2 AND 3)

Dr. Webb is an Assistant Clinical Professor at Duke University. She has over 30 years of diverse nursing practice and leadership experience and has held leadership positions in acute care, behavioral/psychiatric-mental health, home health, and hospice and palliative care. She is a board-certified Hospice and Palliative Care Administrator and a Certified Cultural Intelligence Facilitator and Unconscious Bias Coach. Webb joined the faculty of Duke University School of Nursing in 2020 transitioning to academia from the role of Chief Nursing Officer and Chief Learning Officer for Teleios Collaborative Network. She currently serves as the President-Elect of the Hospice and Palliative Nurses' Association and Hospice and Palliative Nurses Foundation Board of Directors.

ADDITIONAL BOOK RESOURCES

To download a sample chapter and other free book resources, go to http://hdl.handle.net/10755/22481 or scan the QR code below.

TABLE OF CONTENTS

About the Authors.. xi
Contributing Authors.. xv
Additional Book Resources xix
Foreword xxv
Introduction xxvii

1 PRINCIPLES OF CRISIS LEADERSHIP............................1
   Finding Your Footing During the Initial Crisis 2
   Characteristics of the Successful Crisis Leader..................... 3
   Leadership Capacities That Serve Well in Crisis 4
   Key Takeaways.. 17
   Reflective Exercises... 18
   References 21

2 RE-ENVISIONING LEADERSHIP THROUGH THE LENS OF DIVERSITY 23
   Tackling Healthcare Inequity by 2030................................ 24
   Naming Racism in Nursing Leadership 25
   Power and Racism 27
   Nurse Leader Mentor Experience With Race on the Job ... 28
   Authentic Leadership as a Pathway to a More Diverse, Equitable, and Inclusive Nursing Workforce 32
   Unique Leadership Challenges for Historically Marginalized Groups... 33
   Strategies for Developing Leadership Skills 36
   Development and Application of Cultural Intelligence 40
   Key Takeaways.. 41
   Reflective Exercises... 42
   References 46

3 DEVELOPMENT AND APPLICATION OF EMOTIONAL INTELLIGENCE...51
   Emotional Intelligence 52
   Goleman's Model of Emotional Intelligence 53

Emotional Intelligence in Nursing 69
Key Takeaways.. 69
Reflective Exercises... 70
References 73

4 ADAPTABILITY AND DECISION-MAKING 75
Adaptive Leadership... 76
Remodeling Adaptive Leadership 89
Key Takeaways.. 94
Reflective Exercises... 95
References 98

5 CREATIVITY AND INNOVATION IN A TIME OF CRISIS 101
Creation and Innovation in a Crisis................................. 102
Creative Leadership... 105
Creativity Depends on a Solid Foundation 113
Fostering Creativity and Innovation in a Crisis 122
Nursing Innovation in the Covid Era............................. 129
Key Takeaways.. 130
Reflective Exercises... 131
References 133

6 MULTIFACETED COMMUNICATION 135
Communication During Crisis.. 136
The Six Guiding Principles of Crisis Communication 139
The Importance of Reassurance and Transparency.......... 153
Reimagining Communication 155
Key Takeaways.. 158
Reflective Exercises... 159
References 161

7 TEAMWORK AND COLLABORATION 163

- Collaboration and Teamwork: Clarifying Concepts 164
- Coordinating Collaboration During Crisis: The Incident Command System 165
- Foundational Principles for Collaboration 167
- Our Thematic Interviews 170
- Positive Leadership, Motivation, and Mentoring 183
- Working With Teams 186
- Essential Components of Nursing Team Leadership 187
- Key Takeaways 189
- Reflective Exercises 189
- References 191

8 ENSURING CONTINUITY AND STANDARDIZATION DURING RAPID CHANGE 193

- Organizational Continuity 195
- Change Theory During Times of Rapid Modification 198
- Integrating Change in the Middle of the Pandemic 201
- The Need for Standardization 203
- From Preparation to Adaptation 205
- Adaptability and High Reliability Organizations 217
- Nurses Need Organizational Stability 220
- Key Takeaways 223
- Reflective Exercises 224
- References 228

9 COPING, RESILIENCE, AND POSTTRAUMATIC GROWTH 231

- Trauma and Its Outcomes 232
- Deliberate Reflection 237
- Fostering PTG in Organizations 248
- Key Takeaways 251
- Reflective Exercises 252
- References 255

10 NEW BEGINNINGS ... 259
- The Wave Mindset ... 262
- The Secondary Crisis: The Nursing Shortage ... 265
- A New Nursing Leadership ... 266
- Nursing Professional Governance: Structures for Sustaining Nursing Value ... 270
- Change for the Better ... 271
- References ... 274

A STORIES OF LEADERSHIP IN CRISIS ... 277

B ORAL CONSENT SCRIPT FOR A RESEARCH STUDY ... 285

C QUESTIONS FOR MENTOR INTERVIEWS REGARDING CRISIS LEADERSHIP ... 289
- Topical themes ... 290
- Chronological/Sequential (beginning, middle, and end) ... 292

INDEX ... 293

FOREWORD

As time has passed since the first Covid-19 patient was cared for in the US, the experiences of nursing leaders have given us a range of perspectives. Some feel we lost two years of our lives; some question personal adequacy as a leader; and to counterbalance feelings of loss, they all consistently show compassion, courage, and hope. While there have been many times that leaders haven't always known the clear path forward, most have shown elegance, grace, and grit in leading through new experiences. An unexpected encounter with a special nurse helped me take a step forward. Sometime in the last two years, I had the opportunity to talk with a woman, a retired mental health advanced practice nurse who I will call Mrs. N. She was over 100 years old. She was unique in that she had survived the Spanish flu and now had survived Covid. Soon after my time with her, I was to attend the healthcare system Nurse Practice Council, and I asked her what I should say to the nurses. She said, "Be a nurse, don't try to be a doctor when you are a nurse. Doctors and nurses are different, and the world needs nurses."

As I read this book, *Nursing Leadership During Crisis,* it became clear to me how important Mrs. N's message is to leaders—be the leader you are, be real, serve as a leader because the world needs leaders. The methods used by the authors bring clarity as we hear the nurse leaders' voices relate their own accounts of the pandemic. Through the many interviews, the reader can hear the letting go of the tactical, transactional aspects of leadership to reveal their adaptation to the relational aspects. These relational characteristics manifest in leaders as they foster new growth, allow for grace and appreciation, and create a strengthened trust between the nurse and the organization nurses gave so much to support. The gift from this leader transition is the preparation that it provided for the secondary crisis that requires us now to rebuild the nursing workforce.

The second message I received from Mrs. N was this: "Listen to your patients and to each other." The authors make us crave listening. Through their stories, I found myself reflecting over the things we all learned through the pandemic—especially the expectations of the teams we lead—because we listened. This book provides us many answers by assisting the reader in the development of leadership thinking and critical skills by examining the beliefs, actions, and reflections of nurse leaders leading in crises.

As we now consider this current period of thawing that we find ourselves in, we have the opportunity to lead not outside a box but without a box. Let the voices found in this text take us to a place of considering the unique value of nurses and nurse leaders—how will we lead the most trusted profession? Let the voices inform us of how relationships, engagement, and evident nursing contributions are the essence of professional governance. It is also through these relationships that individuals find where they belong. Through this thawing, we must counter the occasional negative perceptions of the practice of nursing that were prevalent through the pandemic. Yes, crises are challenging, and now is the time for leaders to surface the goodness of our profession to show grace and appreciation and foster new growth in our current wave of rebuilding and refinement. How will we now lead so that the practice of professional nursing continues with strong growth in numbers of nurses serving across our great nation? There are many answers to these questions in *Nursing Leadership During Crisis*. Lead with hope and join nurse leaders everywhere as we answer these questions to make sure our cultures are safe, caring, and recognize the humanity in all. Remember, "The world needs nurses."

–Sharon H. Pappas, PhD, RN, NEA-BC, FAAN
Chief Nurse Executive for Emory Healthcare

INTRODUCTION

This book was conceived in the first few months of the pandemic as an attempt to make lemonade out of a deluge of lemons. Just before the first known cases of Covid-19 arrived in the US, 10 nursing students at Emory University had been paired with nurse leader mentors as part of the Leadership Scholars Program (LSP). These LSP students would shadow the mentors over the course of 10 months, build a dynamic network through cohort and mentoring relationships, explore nursing as an integral and leading component of healthcare delivery, and culminate in a leadership project that benefited the nursing mentor's unit or facility.

After matching our students with their mentors in mid-March 2020, Covid forced us to regroup. We began to hear stories from the mentors about the unprecedented leadership challenges they faced during the pandemic. We wondered if we could use our existing partnership between our LSP students with these nurse leaders—not to work on a leadership quality improvement project, as was the original plan, but instead to capture their stories and attempt to understand nursing leadership in crisis.

And thus, over the summer of 2020, we developed a qualitative research proposal, rapidly provided education in qualitative methods and crisis leadership to these LSP students, jointly developed interview questions and the procedures to be followed, received IRB approval, and obtained consent from all mentors. (A copy of the study protocol, verbal consent, and questions asked of the mentors is included in Appendix A, Appendix B, and Appendix C, respectively.) From there, students spent five to six hours conducting interviews with their mentors, transcribed these interviews, and then began the laborious task of evaluation and thematic analysis. Each of us have read, cried over, and laughed with the stories of these true heroes of this pandemic.

We originally set out to capture stories of nursing leaders as they managed the Covid epidemic. Each and every day, nurse leaders were soldiering on against a pathogen that was sickening millions and ending lives. As this book goes to print, the numbers in the US are staggering, with over 97 million sickened and over 1 million dead. Nurses remain at the front line in this battle and sadly represent the majority of the 3,600 healthcare workers who died in the first year of the pandemic (Spencer & Jewett, 2021). This crisis was unlike any that we had ever witnessed in healthcare, and our goal was to give voice to the multitude of daily decisions and actions of leaders of the most trusted profession. However, as we were beginning the process of collecting stories demonstrating unity and collaboration within a profession against a common enemy, as a nation, we were facing divisions, prejudices, and inequities related to race, identity, and social standing. And thus, this book evolved over 18 months to not only discuss leadership in the crisis of a pandemic but also leadership in the crisis of culture that in some ways is more insidious.

The stories and opinions of the nursing leaders we gathered were at times intensely personal and provocative. We struggled with wanting to publicly acknowledge and thank these leaders who graciously shared their lives, opinions, and fabulous insights but at the same time protect their confidences and the facilities they worked for. We publicly can only say how very grateful we are for their time and example, hoping they can recognize themselves in the pseudonyms we settled on to convey a story that is ultimately bigger than all of us. While we started with 10 original student and nurse leader dyads, conversations and recordings often expanded to include other nurse leaders. Some of the best conversations happened in spontaneous focus groups of nurse leaders who shared stories organically, building off of their colleagues. The following table of pseudonyms and collective positions is our best attempt to ascribe the gleanings of these leaders who shared their hearts, minds, and hundreds of years of experience and expertise throughout this book. We will refer to them by these pseudonyms throughout the book to provide an understanding of the role from which they spoke.

Leader Pseudonym	Role Within Organization
Andrew	Chief Quality Officer in Nursing
Rebecca	Director of Nursing Education
Carson	Vice President of Nursing Practice and Education

Amber	Nurse Entrepreneur and Associate Professor
Michelle	Innovation and Advancement Coordinator
Sharma	Director of Nursing Leadership
Kimberly	Nurse Anesthetist and Nursing Faculty
Tanja	Unit Director Labor and Delivery
Symone	Education Coordinator for NICU
Sidney	Federally Qualified Health Center Nursing Director
Kathy	Chief Nursing Officer
Nancy	Critical Care Clinical Nurse Specialist
Jane	Nurse Practitioner Ambulatory Care
Vivian	Critical Care Unit Director

DEFINING NURSING LEADERSHIP

One of the first questions the students asked the nurse leader mentors was, "What is your definition of being a leader?" Recorded in these sessions are personal definitions, anecdotes, and examples.

To understand and reconcile the differences in semantics of the term "leadership," we reached back to our graduate school days and strove to find a concept analysis of nursing leadership. A concept analysis is a formal linguistic exercise to determine meaning, the defining attributes, and characteristics (Risjord, 2009). The basic purpose of concept analysis is to clarify ambiguous concepts in a theory and to propose a precise operational definition that reflects its theoretical base according to recommendations proposed by Walker and Avant (2005). In the most universal of definitions, leadership has been defined by the Oxford English Dictionary (OED) as "the position of a group of people leading or influencing others within a given context; the group itself; the action or influence necessary for the direction or organization of effort in a group undertaking" (OED, 2021a).

"I think a leader recognizes their team, their strengths, what motivates them. A good leader is aware that you don't have to know everything or do everything but recognizes the potential in your team. For example, we have people who teach dysrhythmias, and they are experts. I can't do that. I am just here to support them and make sure they have everything they need to do their best. Also, simply being a good listener. I think being a good leader means that you can be a good follower."

Rebecca, Director of Nursing Education

"I think a part of leadership is vulnerability. We need to be vulnerable. And you need to be flexible. You need to be able to drive a point home but at the same time take feedback and really listen to that feedback, because no one's right all the time. Very rarely are we right most of the time, especially in the time of a crisis when no one knows what is going on. That was a big lesson that I'm still trying to learn is vulnerability—how to be comfortable with that."

Carson, Vice President of Nursing Practice and Education

"[Leadership is] helping to connect the people that work for you with the reasons they do what they do, and then inspiring them to take ownership for those things."

Tanja, Unit Director Labor and Delivery

"It's magic, when you take the time, and when you create a program and a team, not me creating, but together, we're all at the table. When you can be more externally focused and sensitive to everyone within that sphere or system, it sharpens and highlights—for those that do a good job of that and are holistic and democratic in their approach—it highlights what is missing and how it can be done differently. I think a leader that can step into the shoes of a patient . . . who can truly empathize with people's experiences as a healthcare purchaser . . . and, how it feels to be a provider in that setting . . . those are the more effective leaders."

Amber, Nurse Entrepreneur and Associate Professor

"Before the pandemic, I led like the rudder of a boat. If you think about a rudder, it's relatively small compared to the rest of the size of the boat, and the majority of the rudder is underwater, so you don't actually see the rudder when the boat is pulling by. But you know the slightest change in the direction of the rudder drastically changes the direction of the boat. That's the kind of leadership that I aspire to and the leadership that I was trying to practice and build before Covid, to trust my team. I've got an amazing team that I trust. Once Covid hit, I had to take more of a directive approach to leadership command and control at times, just to say we're going to do this now, this has to happen. There's no time for discussion. That's not the best kind of leadership in my opinion. It burns people out quickly; it's not the right way, particularly in nursing, but sometimes you have to do it. So now I think I'm in a hybrid mode depending on what arises. I try to make that decision: What's the leadership approach I need to take for this to do what's best for the team?"

— Carson, Vice President of Nursing Practice and Education

The essence of influencing and inspiring others is the defining element of a leader, regardless of the title. Nursing leadership is in fact replete with multiple levels and titles, from unit supervisor to director, vice president to chief nursing officer. Conferred within these titles are both leadership roles (to inspire and influence) but also managerial functions. In fact, most nurses within management have risen in their ranks because of their specific technical skills, knowledge, and expertise to plan, organize, and coordinate projects and outcomes.

However, purists of management and leadership theory postulate that there are clear and distinct roles that separate a manager from a leader (Zaleznik, 2004). Clearly, as one views any leadership team within a healthcare organization, the frontline supervisors have more management functions, and the leadership team in the C-suite has the responsibility for charting the course of the organization and delegating the operation of the plans to capable subordinates. Yet in healthcare, both are leaders in that they must have a vision and the ability to clearly communicate this vision, lead change, and remain positive and flexible, to name just a few of the traits associated with leadership. For purposes of this book, we are focusing on these leadership characteristics within our identified mentors, regardless of their titled position.

Nearly every list published of the best traits in leaders includes the defining attributes of communication, motivation, delegation, positivity, trustworthiness, creativity, responsibility, commitment, and flexibility. History is similarly replete with examples of effective leaders whose quotes fill this book, and each can serve as a model case. The themes of attributes, the foundational antecedents, and the consequences of leadership traits are the pillars of this book that emerged in the thematic analysis for the 60 hours of interview transcripts recorded between our leadership mentors and the ABSN students. Finally, the *empirical referents*, or measurable aspects of these quantifiable features of interest (Brush et al., 2011), will be explored as chapters within this text.

USING THIS BOOK

"If you don't choose to do it in leadership time up front, you do it in crisis management time down the road."
–Stephen Covey, **management consultant**

Crisis leadership is not a unique entity sprung as a magic charm to save the day. It is built on thoughtful leadership development and foundational elements of structure, established policies and procedures, and trusted communication pathways. While the positions and parent organizations of the nurse leaders we interviewed differed, common thematic elements emerged providing the structure for this book. Each chapter originated as a theme from our qualitative interviews, which we then pursued in literature and media to further substantiate and refine. We often fell back on long-established leadership theories but also pulled from TED Talks, podcasts, internet blogs, and even the musings of leadership consulting firms to provide a synopsis of leadership in crisis that reflects this time. Additionally, we've intentionally brought in other forms of writing throughout this book including plays, historical speeches, quotes from all sorts of leaders, and even publicly available training manuals providing resources but also validating that leadership in nursing is more than just focusing on specific aspects of physical patient care. Nursing is a discipline grounded in liberal arts, and thus an excellent nursing leader liberally assembles their ideology from a multitude of perspectives and disciplines.

We propose that the lessons in this book are best obtained through active and participatory reading and journaling. At the end of each chapter are reflective exercises to assist the reader in carefully considering the concepts presented and then incorporating them into their own leadership meditations. We argue that if a student of leadership will carefully deliberate and explore their beliefs in writing, they will better be able to develop and share their personal philosophy of leadership. Leadership after all is not about project management but is the ability of an individual to influence or guide other individuals, teams, or entire organizations.

One method you will see in each chapter is a format used to structure responses and ideas called the STARR technique (Higgins, 2014). This method has been taught for several years by leadership coaches (Cook, 2009) to assist those interviewing for leadership positions to better present themselves through personal stories. STARR simply stands for:

Situation: Describe the challenging situation.

Task: Describe the task at hand or target desired.

Action: Describe the actions taken and possibly the alternatives available.

Results: Describe the outcome of your actions, including the ability to meet your objective.

Reflection: This extra "R" aims to present your ability to learn and iterate. What did you learn? What would you do differently, the same, or better next time being posed with a similar situation?

We hone our skills when we practice. Similar to muscle memory, we can lay down pathways within our brains through practice. If we consistently use the same approach or pathway in telling a story, we don't have to struggle with what comes next. Like a song, if we know the basic chords or tune of the song, we don't have to struggle with remembering what note comes next. Instead, we can be creative and embellish it with grace notes or slight alterations in the usual rhythm. Develop your storytelling technique by practicing this technique as requested with each topic, first in writing and then through intentional sharing. Soon, you'll have a catalogue of stories to draw from, but more importantly, you'll have such familiarity with this technique that your impromptu stories will be more structured and creative.

A GENTLE JOURNEY FOR THE WEARY

Leaders—during a crisis or even in the everyday—must know who they are, what they know and don't know, what they aspire to be, and what motivates them. We suggest that this book is just one map for a lifelong journey of development and assimilation of attitudes, skills, and behaviors. Writing this book allowed us a therapeutic means to analyze the impact of the pandemic on our personal and professional lives. We believe our discussions with the nurse leaders interviewed also allowed them an opportunity to reflect. And this is exactly what this book will ask of you: to reflect on your leadership development pre-Covid, reflect over your leadership successes and stumbles during Covid, reflect over gleanings from this book, and finally, begin to reflect on the future leader you are becoming.

"Reflect" may be an odd word for the last portion of that sentence. We typically think of reflecting as something that engages looking back; to consider, or meditate—a verb per the Oxford English Dictionary. As used in 1903 by Helen Keller in *Story of My Life* (p. 68): "I used to have time to think, to reflect, my mind and I." And in fact, the beginning and middle directives of that sentence use reflect in exactly that way. But now consider that reflect can also be used figuratively to shed (light) on with rays or beams a subject, question, or issue (sometimes indirectly; OED, 2021b) such as Shakespeare employed with Titus Andronicus (2015/1594, p. 226): "Lord Saturnine: whose virtues will I hope, reflect on Rome as Tytus Raies on earth." We hope that you can reflect some of the learnings and use them to illuminate your path of leadership. The purpose of this book is to assist the reader in developing leadership thinking and critical skills by examining the thinking, actions, and reflections of nurse leaders in crisis. Midway through the book and a good 18 months into our Covid journey, we settled on the title *Nursing Leadership During Crisis: Insights Guiding Leaders From the Covid Pandemic*. We had originally started with a different title, but as you can probably imagine, the title, and even some aspects of this book, evolved as we transitioned from what we originally thought would be a short-term acute crisis to more of a chronic crisis state. As we have done numerous times within these chapters, we felt compelled to re-evaluate perspectives and even challenge conventional thinking and leadership theory down to our choice of words. The title has been no less thought-intensive, being particularly deliberate in choosing the preposition *from*. Clearly, the insights gleaned were during the Covid pandemic, but we also intended that these insights would *lead us away from* this time, *from* this trauma, and *from* the uncertainty that has surrounded all facets of our lives for the past two years. Our hope is that this text will help guide nursing leaders (you!) *from* the Covid pandemic and *to* a mature perspective, integrating theoretical frameworks, ideals, processes, and the reflections of others as you develop your own leadership persona.

REFERENCES

Blair, S. (2020). *10 years to midnight: For urgent global crises in their strategic solutions.* Barrett Koehler.

Brush, B. L., Kirk, K., Gultekin, L., & Baiardi, J. M. (2011). Overcoming: A concept analysis. *Nurse Forum, 46*(3), 160–168. https://doi.org/10.1111/j.1744-6198.2011.00227.x

Cook, S. (2009). *Coaching for high performance: How to develop exceptional results through coaching.* JSTOR.

Higgins, M. (2014, March 10). Using the Star technique to shine at job interviews: A how-to guide. *The Guardian.* https://www.theguardian.com/careers/careers-blog/star-technique-competency-based-interview

Keller, H. (2010/1903). *Story of my life.* Signet Publishing.

Oxford English Dictionary. (2021a). *Leadership.* In Oxford English Dictionary online. https://www.oed.com/

Oxford English Dictionary. (2021b). *Reflect.* In Oxford English Dictionary online. https://www.oed.com/

Northouse, P. (2018). *Leadership: Theory and practice* (8th ed.). Sage Publications.

Risjord, M. (2009). Rethinking concept analysis. *Journal of Advanced Nursing, 65*(3), 684–691. https://doi.org/10.1111/j.1365-2648.2008.04903.x

Shakespeare, W. S. (2015). *The lamentable tragedy of Titus Andronicus.* CreateSpace Independent Publishing Platform. (Original work published 1594.)

Spencer, J., & Jewett, C. (2021, April 8). 12 months of trauma: More than 3,600 US health workers died in Covid's first year. *The Guardian.* https://khn.org/news/article/us-health-workers-deaths-covid-lost-on-the-frontline

Walker, L. O., & Avant, K. C. (2005). *Strategies for theory construction in nursing* (4th ed.). Pearson

Zaleznik, A. (2004, January). Managers and leaders: Are they different? *Harvard Business Review.* https://hbr.org/2004/01/managers-and-leaders-are-they-different

> "Leadership is about making others better as a result of your presence and making sure that impact lasts in your absence."
> –Sheryl Sandberg, former COO, Facebook

1
Principles of Crisis Leadership

The recent Covid-19 pandemic disrupted every aspect of human life—social, political, business, professional, personal, and relational. Unlike the normal and ordinary course of events in our personal and work lives, brutally unusual circumstances like a pandemic catch us by surprise, creating mental, emotional, and physiologic distress. In a crisis, we feel out of control, unclear, multiply challenged, and unsure how to regain equilibrium (Cavaiola & Colford, 2017). It appears as though the rules change dramatically, and the ordinary tools we have for contending with the ongoing events of life no longer seem adequate. We are forced to address new issues that we had not anticipated and are currently beyond our scope of response.

WE ASKED NURSE LEADERS

→ What are the most important qualities for the nurse leader during crisis?

→ What was your internal response during the beginning stages of the Covid crisis in the US?

FINDING YOUR FOOTING DURING THE INITIAL CRISIS

It is the onset of the crisis that creates this immediate disequilibrium. What does not happen, although at times it may feel this way, is the sudden loss of capacity or potential for a viable response to the critical incidents we are confronting. It is the sense of being overwhelmed, immediately challenged, looking for different responses than would have normally emerged in the ordinary course of living one's life or doing one's work.

The leadership skills essential to addressing the elements of a crisis and moving to appropriate response are the same as those expressed in any other leadership situation. In crisis they are merely heightened and intensified, and the timeline for their appropriate exercise is considerably shortened (Johnson, 2018). In addition, the number of leadership skill sets and variabilities diminish to a key few that ascend the leadership hierarchy and take prominence in their utility and viability for immediate problem-solving (Marcus et al., 2019).

There are many different expressions of leadership that nurses, nurse managers, and healthcare organizations use to maintain continuity of care and improve patient outcomes. From the experiences of nurse leaders at all levels, we explore if the leadership approaches required in times of crisis are much different from the leadership expression in normal times. We can be aware that good and accelerated skills in making good judgments are vital during crisis. We also need leadership practices that are best suited for a crisis situation.

While needlessly unilateral during normal times, in a crisis when many difficult decisions need to be made quickly, a more focused leadership approach allows for those decisions to happen quickly and for them to be consistently implemented. Specific examples that have arisen during the pandemic include decisions about what PPE was worn, what lifesaving measures were going to be used, selecting patients for the limited number of ventilators, and who was able to perform or receive elective surgical procedures. These were not easy decisions, and they required justification for the patients and staff members who would be engaged in and affected by those decisions.

CHARACTERISTICS OF THE SUCCESSFUL CRISIS LEADER

The need for more incisive and timebound decisions and actions in a crisis goes without saying. The challenge is to make sure that the connection of the leader with the staff in a professional context is sustained and demonstrates the ownership of decisions and the inclusion of accountable individuals in making them and responding to them. Real-time decision-making and action do not eliminate the need for evidence-based considerations and collective wisdom and the dialogue that actualizes it. Inclusion indicates the leader's responsiveness to the professional staff. This engagement and transparency of both leader and staff lead to better decisions and more sustainable responses. The following elements emphasize the expectations of critical decision-making and team involvement:

- Open to challenging information
- Organized and systemic in preparation
- Responsive to shifts in critical events
- Self-aware regarding readiness and response
- Transparent and vulnerable to self-expression/interaction
- Resilient and determined in the face of challenge
- Confident and trustworthy for others and the organization
- Persistent and patient in steps and stages of addressing crisis

Leadership has no value if something doesn't happen that ultimately leads to making a difference. The behavior of the leader is the best demonstration of the attributes of good leadership. Crisis is a contextual dynamic. It more defines the situation than the subsequent action that is a response to its demands. The individual response of the leader to the crisis sets the frame for how the crisis will unfold and how effective the collective response to it will be. The manifestation of good leader response indicates both the energy and positive character of leaders as they address the specifics of dynamic response. This positive energy transfers to the team, and responding with this positive dynamic sustains the team's engagement as they move through the crisis. Behavioral attributes of the crisis leader include (Pappas et al., 2022):

- Interprets the intensity of the crisis
- Comprehends the meaning of the crisis to people and systems
- Positive attitude, energy, and language directed toward the crisis
- Personal integrity and emotional management of crisis realities
- Communicates frequently at situational and personal level
- Finds critical support emergent leaders in colleagues and teams
- Conceptualizes convergence of issues and responses across crises
- Self-aware and open to personal and team evaluation of role and behaviors
- Adjusts behaviors and responses in face of inadequacies and failures
- Celebrates small tests of change and progress with individuals and teams

Next, we will explore the eight critical skills of crisis leadership that served as the starting point for our qualitative interviews with our nurse leader mentors.

LEADERSHIP CAPACITIES THAT SERVE WELL IN CRISIS

In the March 4, 2020 issue of *Forbes* magazine, leadership contributor Davia Temin, drawing from critical leadership science (Diamond, 2019a; Spector, 2019), pointed out the eight specific leadership capacities that serve us well in a crisis. We used these eight critical skills as the basis for the questions used when interviewing the nurse leaders. (The interview questions can be found in Appendix C.) The eight critical skills are (Temin, 2020):

1. Manage denial.
2. Triage priorities.
3. Solve problems with creativity and innovation.
4. Set clear roles and expectations.
5. Communicate.
6. Provide the information most critical to employee success.
7. Ask for help.
8. Use evidence and emotional intelligence for a broader vision.

Let's take a closer look at each skill.

CRISIS LEADERS MANAGE DENIAL

Of course, one of the first responses to a crisis is disbelief, a kind of certainty that the crisis simply couldn't be true. We also tend to personalize the crisis as though it is specifically happening to us out of context of its impact on anyone else. Building on this foundation, we escalate denial by suggesting that perhaps it's not real, doesn't pertain to me, it will pass, it won't be that harmful, and is likely not as critical as it appears (Diamond, 2019b).

Denial serves an important function. Real or imagined, it provides us a momentary safe space where we can adjust and accommodate to this emerging new reality. Through this accelerated moment in time, we can begin to separate the real data from the fiction. The problem with denial, though, is that if we stay inside of it too long the crisis begins to outpace our response to it, causing missed opportunities to address particularly important issues and time to assess the character and content of the crisis. Unchecked crisis, like a rolling stone, gathers more critical mass as it moves, and the later we address it, the more difficult it becomes to find solutions (Bardon, 2020).

The earliest stages of the crisis provide the best opportunity for assessment. The clearheaded leader, while recognizing the penchant for denial, takes time to sort the real from the fable. Gathering facts as early as possible related to the characteristics and elements driving the crisis helps to provide some early insights into the reality of the crisis in its earliest stages. The more you know and the sooner you know it, the better handle you have on the intensity and trajectory of the crisis and the more likely you are to see potential early actions. Sidney, our FQHC Nurse Director, offered:

> "You always want to see if there is a window of opportunity [while] others may see it as a problem. What can you do to either fix it, change it, or enhance it? Not just sit there, watch it, and talk about it until it spins out of control, because if you do that and go, 'Oh, somebody else can do it,' then you are part of the problem, not part of the solution."
>
> "I don't give up and run away and get mad. Challenge is what I thrive on. I don't look at things that go bad as failure, I look at it as what did I learn from this? What did I learn?"
>
> Sidney, Federally Qualified Health Center Nursing Director

CRISIS LEADERS TRIAGE PRIORITIES

Good leadership response in the middle of a crisis is demonstrated by the person who manages emotional intensity well, works to stay calm and in control, and focuses on the issues. This leader tends to avoid panic and seeks instead to drill down toward a deeper understanding of what's really going on in order to discern some of the early actions that might help to manage the initial stages of the crisis. This leader clearly wants to know what deficits the crisis is creating and what resources are both available and unavailable in beginning to address the crisis. It is at this point that the effective crisis leader begins to look collaterally at others in the workplace, who they may need to communicate and partner with in order to broaden insight, ownership, and engagement of the necessary responses to the crisis and the issues that accompany it. Good crisis leaders know two things about working with others: 1) they cannot resolve the crisis alone; and 2) others will be looking for good leadership in addressing the crisis and when they find it will be willing to lend their skills and resources to address it. Nobody wants the instability a crisis springs. People will generally join their skills and efforts with a good leader who facilitates effective communication and interaction, helping build strong focus in response to each stage of the crisis (Yeboah, 2020).

The effective crisis leader knows that no one can take on all of the crisis issues at once. The leader establishes a pyramid of priorities based on their immediacy and intensity and sorts through them. They then discern those critical priorities upon which responsive goals build or accelerate as a way of removing some of the fuel feeding subsequent and dependent crisis events. Through this concentrated and focused response, the crisis leader "hoses down" some of the early and high-temperature elements of the crisis. By doing so, the leader begins to provide some groundwork to prevent further potential catalysis and begins to build structural and behavioral scaffolding that supports effective and potentially sustainable results. This leader knows that you do today what you can, as much as you can, as fully as you can in the moment. Responding in real time with current real solutions provides the best means and materials to construct the bridge to eventual stability. Finally, if an organization or system has, with any level of readiness, prepared for potential crisis such as the one being currently experienced, it is in its earliest stages that those resources should be accessed. Once the first blush of confusion and panic has passed, the focused leader looks for what plans and resources are available and seeks early access to them (Willink, 2020). It is important, at this stage, to know what tools one has and does not have in order to focus on just what response priorities need to be established and how those priorities are enabled by the preparations and resources in place.

CRISIS LEADERS ARE CREATIVE INNOVATORS

One of the unique characteristics of human survival over the millennia is embedded in the human capacity to adapt. Adaptation equals thriving. Perhaps one of the most useful skill sets for any crisis leader is the capacity to divest ownership of any nonrelevant past practice or processes and to demonstrate a willingness to adjust, create, and invent relevant new ones. Leadership resilience is especially dependent on a high degree of adaptability. Positive engagement alters the perspective from challenge to opportunity. However, due to the crisis, this opportunity is immediate and hits closer to home. Leadership ingenuity in crisis reflects an availability or openness, which creates a goodness-of-fit between crisis-borne challenges and the transformed responses they require (Boni, 2015; McGowen & Shipley, 2020).

Ingenuity and innovation are not unilateral activities. The effective crisis leader recognizes the need to have a collection of the right players in the room, clearly able to engage the crisis and demonstrating a capacity to work effectively together. Gathering the right stakeholders and "setting the right table" for the deliberation, design, and implementation of crisis-addressing strategies is as much an effective leadership behavior in crisis as it is in more ordinary pursuits. The sooner the leader gathers an effective, broad-based crisis team, the earlier they can begin to mitigate the crisis (Weberg & Davidson, 2021).

CRISIS LEADERS SET CLEAR ROLES AND EXPECTATIONS

Gathering the best and the brightest in one space to address a crisis won't have much value if the participants aren't clear about the specific contribution they are there to make. The crisis team as an entity is an important consideration for good crisis leadership. This team serves a specific purpose, grounded in the nature and the action of the crisis and informed by the collective and individual responsibilities for action and resolution that each member of the team brings to the table. In today's work culture, there is likely a highly virtual component of this work team, and structures and strategies of connecting the team and creating an effective structure within which it can work will certainly be first steps. Purpose, roles, functional assignments—along with good decision-making and effective work processes—is the medium through which the effective team operates. The crisis team should not simply be made up of those at the highest levels of leadership in the organization. Indeed, the team should be made up of those who hold relevant knowledge, provide collateral linkages across the system, or are closely related to leadership and workers close to the point-of-work, and are able to accelerate appropriate response. These individuals also have to demonstrate their ability to quickly access relationships, tools, and resources essential to making progress in addressing the crisis. Lacking sufficient time to evaluate competence and effectiveness, short-term judgments about a person's ability to fit into a role and perform it effectively will be an abiding skill set of the leader-facilitator, along with that person's capacity to quickly make personnel and role changes. These changes must be made in a way that advances the opportunity of the team to succeed over the short term; the crisis is not waiting for good leadership alignment (Ferrazzi & Weyrich, 2020).

"At some point you must, even if you feel like you don't have all the pieces or all the answers, you have to make the best decision based on what you know at the time. And you do you have to just go for it . . . We know we've done due diligence—let's pull the trigger. Those are important things. We have brilliant minds at the table, and the discussions and perspectives are rich. Inevitably, you will hear people say something that didn't occur to you, and that's a really good thing. However, you must, as a leader, know when you have gotten enough information, what is actionable, and then *do it.*"

Sharma, Director of Nursing Leadership

CRISIS LEADERS COMMUNICATE

Of course, everyone knows by now that there should always be a crisis plan. However, as everyone also knows, a crisis plan does not generally cover every kind of crisis. Surprisingly, the crisis that arises is often the one for which there has been the least preparation. Still, the elements and components of preparation are generally the same regardless of the crisis. The specifics related to the dynamic of the crisis are the most difficult to plan for, yet make up the majority of the response activities (Centers for Disease Control and Prevention, 2018).

Regardless of the organization's level of crisis preparedness, leadership must be committed to clear, precise, frank, and honest dialogue with all stakeholders. Lies and cover-ups create some of the greatest impediments to collective response to crisis because respondents are often not reacting to the same understanding of the crisis as others and are often working at either inadequate approaches or cross-purposes as they attempt to address their issues of concern (Stewart, 2010). People have a fundamental right to know the truth affecting their lives.

There is much dialogue around the role of leadership related to protecting individuals from the truth because of the pain it may cause them. The logic of this approach is specious. Delaying or attempting to lessen others' pain in the face of an essential yet uncomfortable truth guarantees that when this pain is later fully experienced, its negative intensity and impact will be accelerated (Stewart, 2010). It is the responsibility of the leader to communicate effectively and truthfully. It is the responsibility of those dealing with the truth to own it and act on it. Each having done so, it is also the obligation of the leader to be present to empathize, support, encourage, and enable coping with others' challenges and struggles as they adapt and deal with the truth as it affects their lives. This active support on the part of the leader not only helps others cope with the pain of hurtful information but also enables them to develop insights and personal skills that accelerate their resiliency in the crisis and imbue them with skill sets that help them in successively difficult stages of crisis response (Fearn-Banks, 2017).

Michelle, our Innovation and Advancement Coordinator, described her struggle with honest communication with her staff when those above her were not necessarily forthcoming or transparent with decisions and rationales:

"Folks look at me like, 'Hey you're supposed to be the advocate, what's going on here [with the PPE protocols changing as a result of hospital challenges with decreasing supplies of PPE]?' For me, I don't know, I really don't understand it. Just say we don't have enough [PPE] rather than supply changes are being regulated by what is available based on the demand. I think that we're doing our best but having the message out there that we had enough—I still haven't quite gotten over that, but I will someday. Because I can deal with anything if you're honest. It just didn't sound that way. Even as a leader, I think that that was difficult for other leaders as well."

Michelle, Innovation and Advancement Coordinator

Of course, all of the ordinary and usual principles of effective communication taught in leadership development courses across the world apply just as stringently in crisis events and will not be repeated here. But a final point regarding communication relates to the leader's obligation in crisis situations when they observe how the intensity of crisis response quickly pushes individuals and groups down Maslow's hierarchy. Crisis can drive people to the lowest denominator of ugly human behavior that can result in fracturing the human bond and descending into polarization, compartmentalization, hatred, racism, and a host of other more negative human behaviors (Gold, 2020). At the very earliest stages of crisis confrontation, it is the leader's role to use the tools of positive psychology to remind those who are experiencing negativity of the common bond we have as human beings and of our abiding need to strive with each other as we experience the vagaries and challenges embedded in the crisis (Kleespies, 2017). It is crucial to remind others that the crisis cannot be resolved, and its negative impacts overcome, without the collective positive energy and commitment of all those who are affected by it. In a crisis we truly are "all in this together."

CRISIS LEADERS PROVIDE THE INFORMATION MOST CRITICAL TO EMPLOYEE SUCCESS

All kinds of systems and networks disassemble and fail in a crisis. Because of these breakdowns, false stories, inaccurate scenarios, and misperceptions begin to flow freely between intersections. Stakeholders get caught up in the critical events. It is the conundrum of crisis: When it is critical to have precise and accurate information, less helpful and accurate information is noted. Much of the strings and pieces of data by themselves make no sense and, when woven together, give no indication of right response or true trajectory. It is no help that the media, the internet, cable, and news channels all contribute to the cacophony of conflation and contradiction that often neither edifies nor informs.

The effective critical leader is always looking for multiple sources of information and data as a way of cross-referencing and correlating what they know, finding the points of convergence (Porter-O'Grady & Pappas, 2022). Managing the trajectory of a crisis is often like navigating a storm at sea: There are many forces acting in concert but unfortunately, at times, in opposition to each other, contributing to the disturbance. Sorting through the "noise," digging out inconsistencies, and garnering information that is relevant and useful builds trust and confidence in the words and work of the leader. Furthermore, the leader's tenacious hold on the process of truth-seeking builds confidence and trust in decisions and directions.

Since information is so important to the successful management of crisis, it becomes a tool set for systematic effectiveness (Wagner et al., 2017). Good leaders understand the value of collective wisdom, recognizing that the minds of many provide a resource no one leader, no matter how brilliant, can match. Making sure good information systems and resources are operating in the network provides an infrastructure that allows leadership and responders to stay focused and on a true course. This information infrastructure creates a web of connection that strengthens both collective and unilateral response by assuring that both are operating out of the same general understanding. Even though their roles and responses may be differentiated by their locus and accountability, it is informed by the same reality. The ability to accurately articulate that reality across the system increases the likelihood that synergy will exist in crisis action and response and ultimately aggregate to the benefit of stability for all involved. There is nothing worse in any crisis than the dissonance of well-intentioned actions operating on inadequate or inaccurate information. This chaos multiplies when it occurs in numerous places across the system, each operating off their own information, heading, and direction, contravening the potential for cooperation and integration and ultimately deepening the chaos.

CRISIS LEADERS ASK FOR HELP

Crisis can bring out the best in us. Whether it does so or not is more the product of intentional work than faith or accident. The more emotionally bereft each of us is, the greater the likelihood of drawing inward, pulling one's own close and tight, accelerating the risk of xenophobia and selfishness. All of us are built for survival. While a good instinct, it doesn't arise without disadvantages. Ultimately, one cannot survive in isolation. Human beings are genetically and behaviorally social creatures, depending on each other for their capacity to thrive. Our primordial "fight or flight" DNA can get in the way of this reality regarding our collective ability to thrive.

The effective leader is aware of these dynamics at work, often at cross purposes. A good leader recognizes the need to serve both these dynamics—honoring the need to survive bound up in "fight or flight" and supporting the likelihood to thrive by finding common ground and threading the bonds that bind us to the collective mission of resolving the crisis. This is not an either/or effort. Both urges must be addressed quickly. Definitively assuring individuals and their own are safe and secure provides a firm foundation for moving to conscious and collective action in an intentional concert of broader community response focused on positively addressing the issues. The wise leader is sensitive to the concerns associated with both individual reaction and collective response. Through transparency and vulnerability, the leader connects with the pain and struggles in others, providing a sense of mutual understanding and personal synergy in reacting to the crisis. At the same time, the leader connects the participants to the collective work of response, encouraging them through hope and focus to undertake whatever is necessary to get through the dark moments of the crisis through positive, consistent, and unrelenting response.

None of this leadership work is entirely incidental and responsive. Leadership is a discipline with specific skill sets that distinguish it from other activities. While there are clearly personal attributes that individuals bring to the role that can make them stand out, leadership skills are learned and are the product of scholarly research related to human behavior in the workplace. The exercise of these skills is not about personal traits; it's about the capacity to lead and what one has learned about exercising that leadership (Studer, 2019). Sensitivity to others' struggles and concerns and the facility to enable others to address them are all a part of the positive characteristics of good leadership. Subsequently gathering people together to work in conjunction and collaboration with each other toward crisis resolution is an equally well-defined leadership skill. The requisite for the individual leader is to understand these tenets of good leadership and to have undertaken the disciplines associated with their good exercise. The leader who has done this good work makes all the difference in the world in how a crisis ends.

CRISIS LEADERS USE EVIDENCE AND EMOTIONAL INTELLIGENCE FOR A BROADER VISION

A good leader values knowledge and wisdom. As a species, our development would have gone nowhere if it weren't for our ability to aggregate, collate, and disseminate learning. Good leaders are not only decisive and action-oriented but also learned. We are in this time and place in our world, at this developmental level because of what we've learned and what we've built from that learning.

Effective and sustainable leaders are eager and enthusiastic learners. They are committed to the journey of discernment and discovery; indeed, they are energized by it. Leadership curiosity takes the individual inside the experience of attempting to better understand who people are and how they work. The same is true regarding the leader's curiosity about the world and its workings. This respect for learning scholarship is translated into the effort of good leadership, here again demonstrated by awe and vulnerability (Wilkinson, 2019). This enthusiasm creates a safe space to generalize this energy into the workplace and to make it a subset of the work itself. Enthusiasm for learning in the leader must be palpable so that it becomes a living witness of its value and is more deeply embedded into the culture and life of the workspace.

Enthusiasm for learning also translates into honoring and valuing fact and truth. The wise leader recognizes fact as the accurate discernment of what's real and truth as the journey to that place. Leaders are committed to both and expect this commitment to be a part of the behavioral landscape of the place and the people they lead. As the leader's role is expressed, the sustaining contact with fact and truth remains embedded in the modus operandi of the organization and its people, and formal mechanisms exist to assure that fact and truth remain the operating medium of exchange in the system (McCraw, 2019). Through this process, the leader ensures no compromise of objective fact (the so-called "your facts/my facts") in the search for evidence-grounded truth (as opposed to "truthiness").

A less described part of scholarship is the leader's ability to see immediate issues and concerns in a broader landscape (Weberg et al., 2019)—in short, to see problems from the balcony rather than from the front row. The clue in this scope of vision is the ability to see the links and intersections from the balcony that cannot be clearly seen in relationship to each other while seated in the front row. The ability to solve significant organizational problems is embedded in the facility to see the variety of points of convergence as they impact the whole rather than simply see their operation in key parts of the organization (Porter-O'Grady & Malloch, 2018). The leader's ability to make change is directly related to the breadth of that vision and how it is influenced by the confluence of actions going on concomitantly across the larger system. With this broad systems view, the leader now has sufficient visual scope to translate what needs to happen at the various intersections in the system where more specific applications are needed, yet remain in concert with further related actions needed at other points in the system. This whole-systems view becomes critical to the discernment of problem-solving by the leader no matter at what point of the organization the role is played out.

Finally, as we make the case for the importance of scholarship, we need to add the abiding value of the competencies associated with emotional intelligence. The concept originated by Daniel Goleman (2006) from Harvard University; emotional intelligence includes the three skills of awareness, harnessing, and management of one's own emotions. The discipline of emotional intelligence includes skills related to self-awareness, self-regulation, self-motivation, empathy, and social skills. This package of skills is essentially the tool sets for regulation and expression of one's emotions.

For the manager, it is important to recognize the expressive characteristics of the nurse role as a reflection of the discipline. This discipline is exemplified in understanding the application and expression of the work, the operating relationships in the workplace, the interfacing realities in the work network, and the competencies related to leading others. Because leadership is a discipline, the convergence of each of these elements contributes to the milieu of leadership and to the completeness of its expression. This is especially important in crisis when people and systems are uncertain, disseminating, chaotic, and afraid. The role of the leader in this circumstance becomes a lever in the organization for countering these negative forces with competence, confidence, intelligence, and resilience both functionally and emotionally (Northouse, 2018).

The humanity and humility of good leadership works hand-in-hand with an abiding self-understanding of one's own competencies and challenges (emotional intelligence). Rather than lament their inevitable personal inadequacies, the functional leader looks to supplement and aggregate talent and skills in a way that maximizes their utility regardless of where they may be found (Pink, 2009). Through the convergence of these collective skill sets, the leader can create a positive mosaic of talent that readies the organization for dealing with crisis, creating a collective wisdom that enables creativity and innovation in problem-solving. Through these strategies, complex issues can be better addressed, and the energies and the skills necessary to address their vagaries become more readily available and more useful. In the presence of good crisis leadership, the necessary strategies, responses, skills, and capacity can be harnessed, and a dark present need not stand in the way of a bright future.

CRISIS LEADERSHIP STRUCTURAL TOOLS

Of course, it helps considerably when long-term preparation has readied an organization for inevitable crisis with a well-designed structure for crisis response. Structural tools that should be in place include:

- Preparation management policy utilized
- Crisis command center opened
- Role determination for crisis action
- Priority determination for action
- Specific team role assignment/action
- Resource support system initiated
- Information infrastructure activated
- Action assessment tools initialized
- Communication infrastructure initiated
- Stress reduction mechanisms begun

KEY TAKEAWAYS

In this chapter, we discussed the eight critical skills of crisis leadership as a framework for the questions asked of the leaders interviewed. Because questions can guide answers, it is not surprising that the thematic analysis then revealed a focus on authentic leadership, communication, creativity and innovation, decisiveness, and collaboration.

But before we delve into those areas in the coming chapters, we first need to address the importance of leading change through the lens of diversity, equity, and inclusion. Throughout 2020 and 2021, as a nation and a profession, we have been not only immersed in a battle against a pandemic but also fully engaged in addressing structural, institutional, and personal discrimination based on race, sex, and identity. No discussion on authentic leadership would be complete without addressing how self-awareness, shared vision, and trust are necessary to assure equity and inclusion. Subsequent chapters of this book will discuss strategies and development of leadership skills such as self-efficacy and adaptability, cultural intelligence, and building supportive relationships for inclusive excellence.

REFLECTIVE EXERCISES

1.1 → THE PRIORITIZING PYRAMID

Develop a pyramid of priorities for a professional issue you are struggling with currently. Start by listing out the priorities to the left and then arranging them within the pyramid according to their immediacy and intensity.

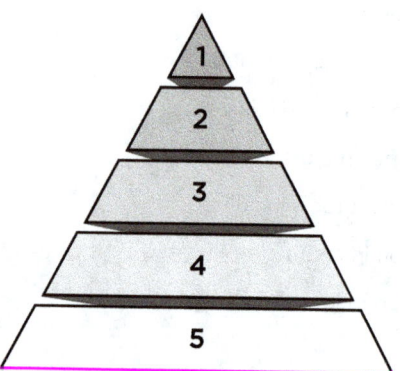

1.2 → REAL-LIFE PRIORITIZATION EXAMPLE

If you had to relocate your patients to a different unit, what would be the first five priorities you would establish to get started?

1. _____
2. _____
3. _____
4. _____
5. _____

1.3 → PERSONAL COMMUNICATION CHALLENGES

When you self-examine your own communication "trip cords," what are the three big triggers that increase feelings of tension within that make you want to stop the communication altogether?

1. _____

2. _____

3. _____

1.4 → SKILL SET ROLE MODELS

Identify by name three colleagues you could count on in a crisis and identify the specific skills/talents they have that you can depend on.

Name	Skill Set

1.5 → AREA OF IMPROVEMENT

Using the STARR technique, describe a specific crisis you faced in your professional life during the pandemic. Then identify the tasks involved, what actions you took, the result of those actions, and what you might do differently in the future.

Situation Describe the challenging situation.	
Task Describe the task at hand or target desired.	
Action Describe the actions taken and possibly the alternatives available.	
Result Describe the outcome of your actions, including the ability to meet your objective.	
Reflection What did you learn? What would you do differently, the same, or better next time being posed with a similar situation?	

REFERENCES

Bardon, A. (2020). *The truth about denial: Bias and self-deception in science, politics, and religion.* Oxford University Press.

Boni, P. (2015). *All hands on deck: Navigating your team through crises, getting your organization unstuck, and emerging victorious.* Career Press.

Cavaiola, A., & Colford, J. (2017). *Crisis intervention: A practical guide.* Sage Publishing.

Centers for Disease Control and Prevention. (2018, January 23). *Emergency preparedness and response.* https://emergency.cdc.gov/cerc/index.asp

Diamond, J. (2019a). *Crisis.* Penguin Random House.

Diamond, J. (2019b). *Upheaval.* Little Brown and Company.

Fearn-Banks, K. (2017). *Crisis communications: A casebook approach* (5th ed.). Routledge.

Ferrazzi, K., & Weyrich, N. (2020). *Leading without authority: How the new power of coal elevation can break down silos, transform teams, and reinvent collaboration.* Random House.

Gold, S. (2020). *Contextual trauma therapy.* American Psychological Association.

Goleman, D. (2006). *Emotional intelligence.* Bantom Books.

Johnson, T. J. (2018). *Crisis leadership: How to lead in times of crisis, threat and uncertainty.* Bloomsbury Business.

Kleespies, P. (2017). *The Oxford handbook of behavioral emergencies and crises.* Oxford University Press.

Marcus, L., McNulty, E., Henderson, J., Dorn, B., & Gergen, D. (2019). *You're it: Crisis, change, and how to lead when it matters most.* Public Affairs, Perseus Books.

McCraw, D. (2019). *Truth in our times: Inside the fight for press freedom in the age of alternative facts.* All Points Books.

McGowen, H., & Shipley, C. (2020). *The adaptation advantage: Let go, learn fast, and thrive in the future of work.* Wiley.

Northouse, P. (2018). *Leadership: Theory and practice* (8th ed.). Sage Publishing.

Pappas, S., Albert, N., Porter-O'Grady T., & Malloch, K. (2022). *Quantum leadership: Creating sustainable value in health care.* Jones and Bartlett.

Pink, D. (2009). *Drive: The surprising truth of what motivates us.* Canongate.

Porter-O'Grady, T., & Malloch, K. (2018). *Quantum leadership: Creating sustainable value in health care* (5th ed.). Jones & Bartlett.

Porter-O'Grady, T., & Pappas, S. (2022). Professional governance in a time of crisis. *Journal of Nursing Administration, 52*(4), 217–224. https://doi.org/10.1097/nna.0000000000001134

Spector, B. (2019). *Constructing crisis: Leaders, crises, and claims of urgency.* Cambridge University Press.

Stewart, R. S. (2010). Telling patients the truth. *The Online Journal of Health Ethics, 6*(1), 1–10.

Studer, Q. (2019). *The busy leader's handbook: How to lead people and places that thrive.* Wiley.

Temin, D. (2020, March 4). Crisis leadership in real time: 8 pandemic best practices. *Forbes.* https://www.forbes.com/sites/daviatemin/2020/03/04/crisis-leadership-in-real-time-8-pandemic-best-practices/#72fbfc59797e

Wagner, K., Lee, F., & Glaser, J. (2017). *Healthcare information systems: A practical approach for healthcare management.* Jossey Bass.

Weberg, D., & Davidson, S. (2021). *Leadership for evidence-based innovation in nursing and health professions.* Jones & Bartlett.

Weberg, D., Mangold, K., Porter-O'Grady, T., & Malloch, K. (2019). *Leadership in nursing practice.* Jones & Bartlett.

Wilkinson, H. (2019). *Learners as leaders.* Bibliolife, LLC.

Willink, J. (2020). *Leadership strategy and tactics.* St. Martin's Press.

Yeboah, C. (2020). *Succeeding in times of crisis.* Independently published.

> "The beauty of anti-racism is that you don't have to pretend to be free of racism to be anti-racist. Anti-racism is the commitment to fight racism wherever you find it, including in yourself. And it's the only way forward."
> –Ijoema Oluo, author

2

Re-envisioning Leadership Through the Lens of Diversity

Given the unprecedented time of a global pandemic that has unmasked long-standing racial and ethnic disparities and changing US demographics, diversifying the nursing workforce and nursing leadership has become a high priority. However, the lack of diverse representation in nursing is profound and does not resemble the increasingly diverse America (Sullivan Commission, 2004). The year 2020 marked a decade of change in the US racial composition. The nation became more racially and ethnically diverse, with gains in nearly all categories of race except whites, which declined to 57.8% from 63.7% (US Census Bureau, 2021).

WE ASKED NURSE LEADERS

→ Considering your experiences, what challenges have you encountered when you have led a team from diverse racial and ethnic backgrounds during crisis (e.g., nursing shortage, Covid-19 response)?

→ How have you or your organization addressed inequities and injustices in the workplace?

While the country experienced a shift in racial demographics, representation of nurses from historically underrepresented groups remains low, at 19.2% of the registered nurse workforce (American Association of Colleges of Nursing [AACN], 2019). The AACN (2019) also reported that in 2017, white registered nurses represented 80.8% of all registered nurses in the US, indicating that less than 20% of the workforce were represented by nurses of color.

TACKLING HEALTHCARE INEQUITY BY 2030

The racial and ethnic discordance between US demographics and nursing representation has led to national calls for expansive efforts to diversify the nursing workforce. These deliberate aims are viewed as a critical part of the solution to address long-standing health inequities among underrepresented groups (National Academy of Medicine [NAM], 2021), the same population that has experienced significant growth in the US.

Considering the complexities in healthcare, historical legacies, and renewed commitments to expanding diversity within the profession to advance health equity, the question that emerges is: Who will respond in leading the charge in nursing? To fully actualize these goals, nursing leaders must acknowledge the harmful effects of racism within the profession and the crucial importance of diversity, equity, and inclusion (DEI) to drive progress toward health equity (NAM, 2021).

As the faces of the nation are changing in racial and ethnic composition, nurses are expected to possess knowledge, expertise, and competencies in the provision of culturally congruent care across the continuum and address racism in system-based practices (AACN, 2021; NAM, 2021). During this time of social relevance, nurse leaders are required to understand the intersectionality of health, racism, and discrimination based on gender identity, sexual orientation, geographic residence, and circumstances associated with ability and mental health conditions (NAM, 2021). Nurse leaders must also move beyond acknowledgment and understanding to meaningful actions that contribute to actualizing DEI goals.

For nurses to lead in evolving healthcare systems and meet current and future demands to diversify the profession, new leadership approaches within the discipline will be necessary. While the number of nurses of color (NOC) in the workforce is low, diverse representation in nursing leadership is even lower (Waite & Nardi, 2017). According to the American College of Healthcare Executives, only 16% of C-suites executives within the highest leadership rank in US hospitals are racially diverse (Bowen, 2020). In nursing, the percentage of deans and nurse executives from historically underrepresented groups is significantly low, representing less than 6% overall (American Nurse Association [ANA], 2021; Iheduru-Anderson et al., 2021). These racial disparities in nursing leadership are a symptom of deeper problems that are often not openly discussed and thus continue to perpetuate the deeply embedded thorns of racism (Iheduru-Anderson et al., 2021).

NAMING RACISM IN NURSING LEADERSHIP

Leading change in healthcare environments that are propelled by DEI goals is a unique opportunity for nursing. However, the pernicious influence of racism that has shaped American history poses the greatest threat to reaching these ideals. Naming racism and recognizing the systemic and generational impact it has in healthcare, wealth distribution, economic viability, hierarchal structures, and educational and career opportunities encourages authentic dialogue in the profession that creates a shift toward racial and social justice (Iheduru-Anderson, 2020; Villarruel & Broome, 2020; Walter et al., 2017). The *Future of Nursing 2020–2030* report calls for nurse leaders to acknowledge the historical context of racial inequities in nursing and the role they must assume to address and dismantle all forms of racism and discrimination to build a diversified nursing workforce (NAM, 2021).

> ## RACE, RACISM, AND DISCRIMINATION: WHAT DO THESE TERMS REALLY MEAN?
>
> **Race:** A social construct that is used as a social marker to describe a group of humans based on physical traits associated with shared ancestry (Flanagin et al., 2021).
>
> **Racism:** An organized social system, established by the dominant group, that ranks individuals into social groups that are considered inferior. The dominant group exerts its power to devalue and disempower other racial groups (Williams et al., 2019).
>
> **Structural racism:** A form of racism that provides advantages to the dominant group while disadvantaging and oppressing or neglecting other racial groups. Structural racism is associated with residential segregation and disparities in education attainment, employment status, incarceration rates, fatal police shootings, and judicial treatment (Williams et al., 2019).
>
> **Cultural racism:** Belief in inferiority of values, language, symbols, and assumptions of the larger society. Cultural racism is where negative stereotypes and implicit bias about a race are created and internalized (Williams et al., 2019).
>
> **Discrimination:** A form of racism that is expressed in treating racial groups differently. These differences result in inequitable access to resources and opportunities (Williams et al., 2019).

The National Commission to Address Racism in Nursing reports that NOC have been on the receiving end of unfair structural employment practices and processes across work settings (ANA, 2020, 2021). This further substantiates the evidence showing that the low representation of NOC in executive positions is a consequence of the long-standing institutional inequities and racism in the profession and healthcare systems. Historically, dialogue in nursing has typically not included racism, oppression, and privilege (Iheduru-Anderson, 2020), but the many injustices that have been underscored during these unprecedented times have confirmed that it is necessary and long overdue. The National Commission to Address Racism in Nursing report indicates that failure to acknowledge and address racism in nursing may result in moral and physical harm. Inactions impact NOC and hinder entry, practice, and research and leadership roles in nursing (ANA, 2021). For example, the Covid-19 pandemic unveiled many inequities in the disproportionate burden of disease among people of color (POC) but also revealed inequities within the profession. Among 10,000 nurses, the 2020 American Nurses Foundation New Pulse on the Nation's Nurses Survey showed that Black and Hispanic/Latino nurses were two times more likely to be diagnosed with Covid-19 than white nurses (ANA, 2020). It was also noted that disproportionate numbers of Black and Hispanic/Latino nurses were represented on the front line caring for patients with Covid compared to white nurses: 58%, 63%, and 49% respectively (ANA, 2020).

There have been several expressions of racism that have diminished the presence of NOC. Beard and Julion (2016) conducted a study on the experiences of African American faculty participants, who indicated that they often experienced racism and discrimination. Faculty attributed skin color to negative stereotypes and perceptions of being less intelligent (Beard & Julion, 2016). Other findings suggest that compensation disparities, intentional exclusion, and additional expressions of racism affect the success of NOC (Beard & Julion, 2016; Evans, 2013). The invisibility of racism and its effects cannot be overstated, as it has also been attributed to hiring and promotion inequities and barriers to entry into leadership positions (Beard & Julion, 2016; Beard et al., 2020).

POWER AND RACISM

Is power good or bad, or does that depend on how it's used? Power is dynamic and can be used to advance organizational goals and priorities. The power structures within organizations determine who participates in decision-making, as well as the diverse representation within positional authority that can advance DEI goals (Simonsen & Shim, 2019). Power can be leveraged to propel teams to achieve organizational goals and should be shared among all racial and ethnic groups at all levels in institutions (Sullivan Commission, 2004; VeneKlasen & Miller, 2002).

However, power differentials within healthcare organizations and academic institutions are important factors that, if abused, can stifle potential growth and contribute to racist practices and attitudes in nursing that influence leadership opportunities and how leadership operates.

Power is multidimensional and complex, and when expressed as domination, resistance, and lack of collaboration, it is exploitative (Guinaran et al., 2021). *Power over* is a concept associated with discrimination, corruption, and abuse and describes how power is used to control and prevent others from acquiring it. Exercising *power over* is challenging because it often does not operate in visible forms (VeneKlasen & Miller, 2002).

Power is a key driver in racial inequities and explains how some individuals manage and control influence, information, and resources within institutions. There are three interactive dimensions of power (Nardi et al., 2020; VeneKlasen & Miller, 2002):

1. *Invisible power*, where problems and issues are not disclosed at the decision-making table, and information is withheld from certain individuals
2. *Hidden power* involves controlling the agenda at the decision-making table and selecting who is invited
3. *Visible power* shapes formal rules, structures, authorities, and decision-making processes

These forms of power influence control of communication, exclusion, misinformation, powerlessness, and biased policies and practices (VeneKlasen & Miller, 2002).

NURSE LEADER MENTOR EXPERIENCE WITH RACE ON THE JOB

In listening time and again to the interviews conducted with our nurse leaders, we were surprised to not hear any mention of injustice or inequity because of race, gender, or sexual identification, nor concerns about lack of diversity in healthcare or within the various leadership levels. The cohort of mentors themselves, while largely female, included three who identified as POC and two who identified as male.

Only Carson, the Vice President of Nursing Practice and Education, discussed the social inequity when directly questioned:

"So it's definitely been challenging, but I think what has helped me is having a really solid network of support and resources, because literally it feels like every day it's something, whether it's Covid or whether it's social injustices or systemic racism. With the police brutality, it just felt like 'Oh my God' every single day. But I think having people that you can talk to who can be a sounding board and having leaders who are deeply committed to social justice and don't mince words are important for me. So now I work for an organization that's not perfect but really takes a solid stand on what is right, what is just, and what will not be tolerated. And is also transparent enough to recognize the areas where we could do a little bit better. So that has helped me tremendously, you know, to be able to come to work and share with my own boss, 'After the news last night I am not OK.' I'll tell you at least for me personally I have a great deal of confidence in the strength of our nurses and their clinical competence in their ability to care for almost any complex patient situation. But the social injustices compounded everything else that we were dealing with, and that was for me what felt especially overwhelming."

Carson, Vice President of Nursing Practice and Education

Worried that we might have missed an important topic in our interviews conducted in the summer and fall of 2020, we went back to our leaders in the fall of 2021 with a short set of follow-up questions specific for DEI. We asked the following questions directly:

- Did they face elements of racism, inequity, or injustice as leaders in their respective healthcare organizations?

- Were they aware of any unjust or discriminatory practices?
- Did leading during a pandemic that coexisted with a time of social unrest, issues around police brutality, and racial injustice affect them personally or professionally?

We were surprised that seven out of the eight leaders who agreed to be re-interviewed answered with affirmations that their organization had solved those issues years ago. While these leaders were from separate entities and parent companies, most were quick to deny any racial injustice and felt their healthcare facilities did a great job with promoting diversity and inclusion.

As previously noted, only Carson recognized diversity and equity as a continued major issue. He offered:

> "One thing that our healthcare organization has not done but is doing a better job at, and we have a long way to go, is how we address racial injustice and inequity within our health system. We have a lot of gaps, a lot of pieces we can do a better job at. I'm glad that we are finally talking about it, but I think that action is needed in addition to talk."
>
> Carson, Vice President of Nursing Practice and Education

We shared with Carson that he was the only leader who felt that more gains were needed in terms of equity and inclusion in healthcare leadership. He was quick with figures and a perspective that explained the previous voices:

"When I think about leadership, currently to date, roughly 70% of our healthcare staff comes from an underrepresented population. Our leadership is not near that. Our nurses should look like the community they serve, and leadership should be the same. The racial inequity and injustice is an ongoing concern that will take generations to get to where we need to go. It's an important question to ask, and for leaders to look at. There is a lot of reactionism, a lot of white fragility, and a lot of people refusing to look at their upbringing, background, privilege, and experience for fear that they might feel something [uncomfortable]. That refusal to look at it, especially within the leadership team, is a detriment."

Carson, Vice President of Nursing Practice and Education

Finally, he went on to propose that the leaders we had previously interviewed were too distant from the situation, too removed:

"People are so separated and distanced from it. In *Just Mercy* by Bryan Stevenson, he talks about this concept of proximity that the people closest to the problem are closest to the solution. I think that is a huge flaw in healthcare leadership. Leaders are so removed: They wear business dress, have big titles, [but] we are so distant from what is actually happening. Sadly, we have a lot of people leaving because of it, and they are not comfortable telling why they are leaving."

Carson, Vice President of Nursing Practice and Education

AUTHENTIC LEADERSHIP AS A PATHWAY TO A MORE DIVERSE, EQUITABLE, AND INCLUSIVE NURSING WORKFORCE

As the profession moves forward into the mid-21st century, we enter a new epoch that requires resilient, diverse, and *authentic* leadership. Authentic leaders possess distinguishing characteristics and engage in specific leadership behaviors that can enhance and accelerate the journey to a diverse, equitable, and inclusive nursing practice environment.

While there are many different leadership theories and styles of leadership, authentic leadership may be used with any other leadership style to exert a positive organizational influence (Johnson, 2019).

Authentic leadership theory is a complex theory borrowing largely from humanistic psychology, which emphasizes the role of self-awareness, self-mastery, and "the quality of being real or true" (Cambridge Dictionary, n.d.). Fundamental to authentic leadership is the belief that humans are the most important organizational asset. Authentic leaders promote an ethos of purposeful and value-driven leadership where characteristics such as self-discipline, transparency, and *leading with the heart* are displayed. The theory has been widely researched in nursing and healthcare administration and is associated with numerous positive attitudinal changes and behavioral outcomes that enhance job performance, collaboration, and staff retention. Other organizational benefits include commitment, engendered trust in the leader, loyalty, and increased motivation (Alilyyani et al., 2018).

Authentic leaders inspire a shared vision for healthy, diverse, and equitable workplaces. Safe, high-quality care results from building relationships where transparency, openness, and honest communication is the norm. These values and attributes are critical for building a culture of trust, effective teamwork, and excellence in interprofessional collaborative practice.

UNIQUE LEADERSHIP CHALLENGES FOR HISTORICALLY MARGINALIZED GROUPS

Leading with authenticity is a developmental journey that demands a commitment to never-ending self-discovery and self-awareness. It requires a willingness to reflect on personal strengths, weaknesses, biases, and needs for growth and development. Authentic leaders develop in psychologically safe environments that exude an atmosphere of trust, support, and constructive learning and development (Frazier et al., 2017; Fujimoto & Presbitero, 2021). This environment dispels fear, allows risk-taking, fosters genuine self-expression, and allows space to learn from leadership mistakes and to identify opportunities for improvement.

All leaders experience challenges as they develop in their roles as leaders, yet nurses from historically marginalized groups experience additional unique challenges often resultant from factors beyond their control. These factors often include identity-related characteristics, such as race/ethnicity, nationality, gender, age, and others (Fowler, 2020). The enduring legacy of racism in nursing has led to a persistent scarcity of diverse representation of leadership within organizations and academic institutions. The pervasive effects of structural and systemic racism limit access to leadership positions, development, and promotional opportunities. Isolation, discrimination, and biases, which are corollaries of racism (Fowler, 2020), also inhibit certain attributes of authentic leaders, including open expression of vulnerability and willingness to take chances in decision-making.

CODE-SWITCHING: WHO IS SHOWING UP?

One of the practices among nurses from historically marginalized groups (HMGs) that stifle the development of authentic leaders is code-switching, a practice used by individuals from HMGs where there are prevailing stereotypes and biases (McCluney et al., 2019). *Code-switching* is a conscious or subconscious adjustment made in expression, behavior, speech, manner, and physical appearance to accommodate others to increase the chances of fair treatment, quality service, and employment opportunities. Individuals from any race, ethnicity, or gender may code-switch to gain acceptance and respect within dominant groups.

Conventionally, code-switching has a linguistic context and has been used to describe the seamless switching between two or more languages by bilingual and multilingual individuals. However, code-switching has context that extends beyond language and denotes behaviors and expressions used to fit in a sociocultural norm and/or to avoid the harmful effects of negative stereotypes and biases that are often experienced by HMGs in the workplace (McCluney et al., 2019).

The degree to which nurses from HMGs code-switch is further influenced by the effects of power relations. Possessing or lacking power within an organization contributes to how code-switching is directed. Oftentimes, it is directed towards acceptance from individuals in positions of power for professional survival and validation (McCluney et al., 2019).

Evidence suggests that Black and Hispanic people code-switch at higher rates than white people (Anderson, 2019; Dunn, 2019). In a Pew study, 57% of Black respondents reported that their racial background hindered their ability for career growth. Black respondents perceived that their intelligence was often questioned, and racial discrimination negatively impacted their fair treatment in employment, salary, and career advancement (Anderson, 2019). These findings may explain why nurses from HMGs code-switch in health systems and academic institutions.

Code-switching practices can serve as barriers to leadership advancement for nurses from HMGs and impede their ability to lead authentically (Godsil et al., 2014). When personal and professional identity cannot coexist in the workplace because of racism and classism, mental health exhaustion and burnout can ensue. The lack of integrating both identities can lead to cognitive depletion and underperformance (McCluney et al., 2019).

Code-switching creates a conflict between self-expression and social acceptance whereby individuals take on one identity in environments where there is no fear or threat to being authentic (i.e., at home) and another in environments where there is perceived threat (i.e., at work). Switching from and suppression of the authentic self to the socially accepted self requires a significant expenditure of energy and results in emotional exhaustion. Additionally, lower self-esteem can develop from the suppression of the authentic self and the internal conflict of code-switching (McCluney et al., 2019).

Conventional environments may include organizational systems whose cultures are centered on whiteness as the norm. Organizations have historically operated under the guise of being equal opportunity employers, yet, due to gaps in awareness and acknowledgment, fail to create a milieu of equity, inclusion, and belonging for HMGs. Nurses who have non-English or non-European accents may attempt to tone down, mask, or "cover" their accents so that they "fit in" and to avoid perceptions of inferiority (Chakraborty, 2017; Shah, 2019). Similarly, the intellectual aptitude of nurses who are English language learners has been called into question, and these nurses have frequently been overlooked for leadership and other highly sought-after positions because of their vernacular (Giles & Coupland, 1991; Shah, 2019).

COVERING

Covering, much like code-switching, is a corollary practice that individuals from HMGs use to garner acceptance and, most significantly, employ it as a defense mechanism in the face of discrimination, ridicule, and racism. Erving Goffman (1963) defines *covering* as downplaying identity traits—such as religious affiliations, sexual orientation, gender, ethnicity, socioeconomic status, etc.—to assimilate into conventional environments (Goffman, 1963). Kenji Yoshino (2006) further developed the concept of "covering." He identified four categories of covering (see Figure 2.1):

- **Appearance:** Altering expression to fit in (e.g., physical presentation style, hair style)

- **Association:** Distancing self from members of affinity group

- **Affiliation:** Evading aspects of identity aligned with negative stereotypes that are often assigned to certain groups

- **Advocacy:** Degree to which one defends the group(s) to which they belong.

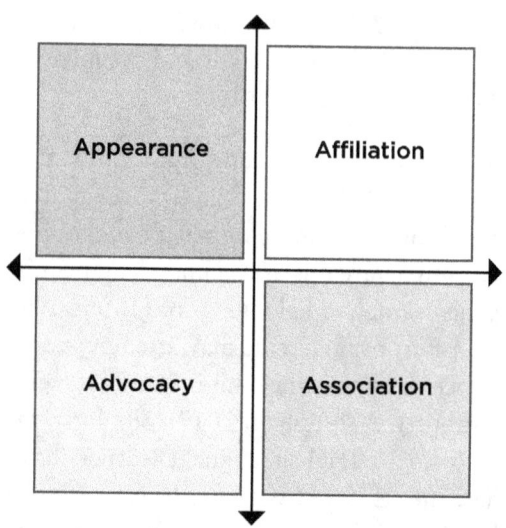

FIGURE 2.1 Four axes of covering (Smith & Yoshino, 2019).

STRATEGIES FOR DEVELOPING LEADERSHIP SKILLS

The role of a leader comes with immense accountability and responsibility that requires specific skills for ongoing growth and promoting development of diversified teams. Adaptability and self-efficacy are two essential skills that leaders need to establish and maintain organizational well-being from a personnel perspective and for the success of the organization. However, development of these skills may be difficult without specific strategies. Effective mentoring, emotional intelligence, and cultural intelligence are symbiotic. Each concept is empirical and grounded in evidence-based frameworks that enrich the ability to lead through a global lens. Within this chapter we will conclude with two of these strategies—mentoring and cultural intelligence—before diving deep into the concept of emotional intelligence in Chapter 3.

THE IMPORTANCE OF MENTORING

Leadership development and career advancement of nurses from HMGs are important to build a culturally diverse and equitable nursing workforce. A key strategy to developing and supporting successful nurse leaders from HMGs is mentoring. *Mentoring* implies a purposeful creation of a relationship between an experienced nurse who shares their knowledge, expertise, and lived experience with a less experienced nurse who seeks personal and professional growth and development (Matza et al., 2018; Moore & Wang, 2017). The mentoring relationship is based on mutual respect, trust, and appreciation of individuality (Matza et al., 2018). Mentoring involves respect, trust, formulating goals around continuous learning, career advancement, engagement, and succession planning (Jakubik et al., 2017).

Many models of mentorship exist, yet the best approaches are those that are based on a comprehensive and culturally sensitive appraisal of the needs of the mentee that informs an individualized mentorship plan. One such mentoring model is the *mutual exchange model of reciprocal mentoring,* in which both individuals reciprocate the role of mentor and mentee so that there is an even exchange in terms of understanding each other from a cultural perspective (Desai et al., 2018). This type of mentoring facilitates a professional development approach that takes individual cultures into account and supports diversity and inclusive excellence. For nurse leaders or nurses from HMGs aspiring to become leaders, consideration must be given to garnering resources within and external to the organization to meet the unique mentoring needs arising from the extant lack of adequate diversity in the profession.

SIX MENTORING PRACTICES

Jakubik et al. (2016a) outline six mentoring practices and associated benefits to achieve mentoring goals that can be used in developing nurse leaders from HMGs (see Figure 2.2). The mentoring activities are flexible and informed by the partnership between the mentor and mentee. The activities should be modified based on the needs of the organization and at the discretion of the mentor and mentee. Mentoring practices include (Jakubik et al., 2016a):

- Welcoming
- Mapping the future
- Teaching the job

- Transitional support
- Protection
- Leadership development

WELCOMING

Welcoming, the first of the practices, focuses on introduction to the workplace, understanding organizational norms, and activities that lead to a sense of belonging (Jakubik et al., 2016b). Sense of belonging can only exist if the mentors and mentees are allowed to be their authentic selves (Rattan, 2021) and to be valued by each other, the leadership team, and the organization.

MAPPING

Mapping the future is the second mentoring practice that leads to career optimism. Role-modeling, career planning, and setting SMART (Specific, Measurable, Achievable, Realistic, and Time-Bound) goals are directed at future-oriented outcomes (Jakubik et al., 2016c). Application of this mentoring practice helps to prepare the mentees for future career opportunities, including those made available as part of the organizational succession plan.

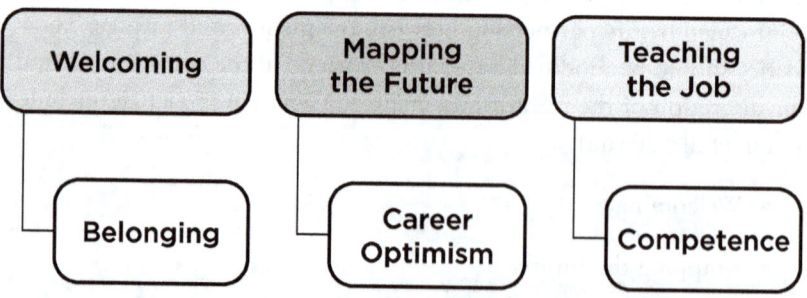

FIGURE 2.2 Six mentoring practices and benefits.

TEACHING THE JOB

Teaching the job is the third mentoring practice and leads to competence and confidence in performing the new role. Mentors share their expertise to educate and promote essential skills development (Eliades et al., 2017).

SUPPORTING THE TRANSITION

Supporting the transition is a practice approach that mentors use to advance growth and confidence through development of communication, decision-making, and problem-solving skills (Jakubik et al., 2016d).

PROTECTION

Protection is the fifth mentoring practice that leads to psychological safety and security. The mentors provide a psychologically safe environment where the mentees feel comfortable sharing their mistakes (Jakubik et al., 2016e).

LEADERSHIP DEVELOPMENT

The final mentoring practice is the preparation for leadership that focuses on developing specific management and leadership competencies. This is critical to leadership roles at all levels and includes succession planning within the organization. The mentors explore learning experiences that facilitate the mentees' leadership skills as they become agents of change within the organization and feel confident to take risks (Jakubik et al., 2017).

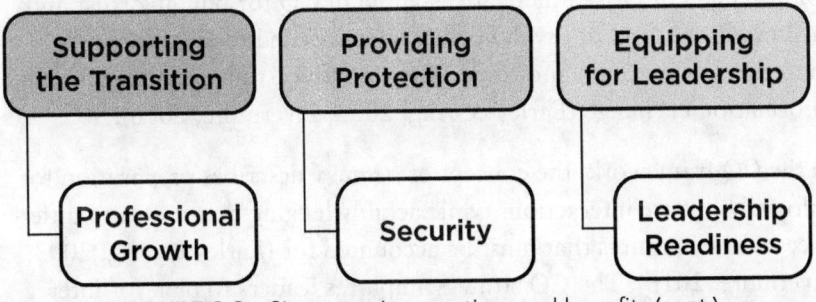

FIGURE 2.2 Six mentoring practices and benefits (cont.).

DEVELOPMENT AND APPLICATION OF CULTURAL INTELLIGENCE

Cultural intelligence (CQ) is a research-based framework that is used to acquire the skills and confidence to navigate multicultural environments (Earley & Ang, 2003). There are four capabilities required to develop CQ (Earley & Ang, 2003; Livermore, 2016):

1. Motivation
2. Knowledge
3. Strategy
4. Action

Motivation describes individual levels of enthusiasm about interacting with people from different cultures (Earley & Ang, 2003; Livermore, 2016). Leaders who prioritize diversity are intrinsically driven to create teams that are representative of multiple cultures because they recognize the benefits of diverse lived experiences (Livermore, 2011, 2015, 2016).

The CQ capability of *knowledge* applies to not only gathering information that focuses on what people have in common but also seeking to learn more about cultural differences (Earley & Ang, 2003; Livermore, 2016). Operationalizing this capability could be shown by leaders who are intentional in forging authentic relationships through intimate interactions focused on really getting to know individuals within organizations. In the next chapter, we'll take a deep dive into emotional intelligence (EI) as an essential tool in crisis leadership. Many of the EI competencies discussed there are essential in CQ for building trust and facilitating the level of psychological safety needed to create an environment that supports and respects vulnerability, thus enabling specific information exchange (Earley & Ang, 2003; Livermore, 2016).

In the CQ framework, the concept of *strategy* describes preparation for culturally diverse interactions while acknowledging that there are differences within cultures that must be accounted for (Earley & Ang, 2003; Livermore, 2016). The CQ strategy implores leaders to plan for interactions with individuals and groups from other cultures without imposing norms, generalizations, and stereotypes.

The final CQ capability, *action*, refers to flexibility and adaptability during multicultural collaborations (Earley & Ang, 2003; Livermore, 2016). As a component of the CQ framework, action describes behaviors that require EI and assist in compromise (Livermore, 2016). Application of the four CQ capabilities in tandem helps leaders to appreciate the advantages of diversity teams beyond demographic characteristics and metrics.

> **ADDITIONAL LEARNING**
>
> **Listen:** AT&T's Anne Chow: *Creating a Safe Workplace:* https://hbr.org/podcast/2021/06/ats-anne-chow-creating-a-safe-workplace
>
> **Read:** *A New Prescription for Power:* https://hbr.org/2020/07/a-new-prescription-for-power

KEY TAKEAWAYS

Authentic leadership and practices will enable nurse leaders to overcome challenges, continue to advance the profession, and ensure it fulfills its role in transforming the healthcare system and advancing health equity. To do so requires intentional and ongoing engagement in specific professional and personal development endeavors. Two of the three pivotal strategies for expanding leadership skills and developing future leaders who embrace the significance of diversity among teams were presented in this chapter: mentorship and CQ. These skills are important for leaders and all members of organizations. Nurse leaders must prioritize inclusive excellence through targeted recruitment and retention of nurses from historically underrepresented and marginalized populations to build a diversified workforce.

REFLECTIVE EXERCISES

2.1 → PERSONAL EXPERIENCES OF COVERING

Identify the forms of covering you have engaged in or observed. In the space to the right, write specific examples.

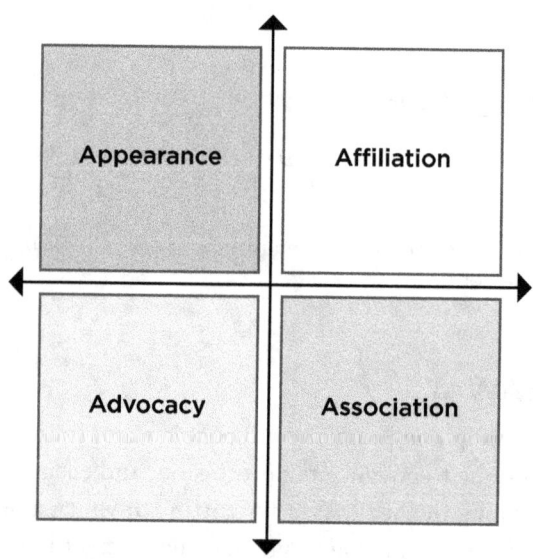

2.2 → FIRST AWARENESS OF RACE

Using the STARR technique, describe the first time in your professional life when you were involved in an issue surrounding racial inequity. You might not have handled this situation as you would today, but regardless, complete the table and develop your narrative. How did you feel, think, and interpret the experience? If you are white, also reflect on how you think this differs from your Black and/or POC colleagues.

Situation Describe the challenging situation.	
Task Describe the task at hand or target desired.	
Action Describe the actions taken and possibly the alternatives available.	
Result Describe the outcome of your actions, including the ability to meet your objective.	
Reflection What did you learn? What would you do differently, the same, or better next time being posed with a similar situation?	

2.3 → PERSONS OF INFLUENCE

Construct a diagram and place yourself in the middle. Create additional shapes around the center shape (reflecting yourself) with lines of influence. In those external shapes, identify the persons of influence (PI) who have the power to impact your career success and advancement. Examine your relationship with those individuals and ask the following questions:

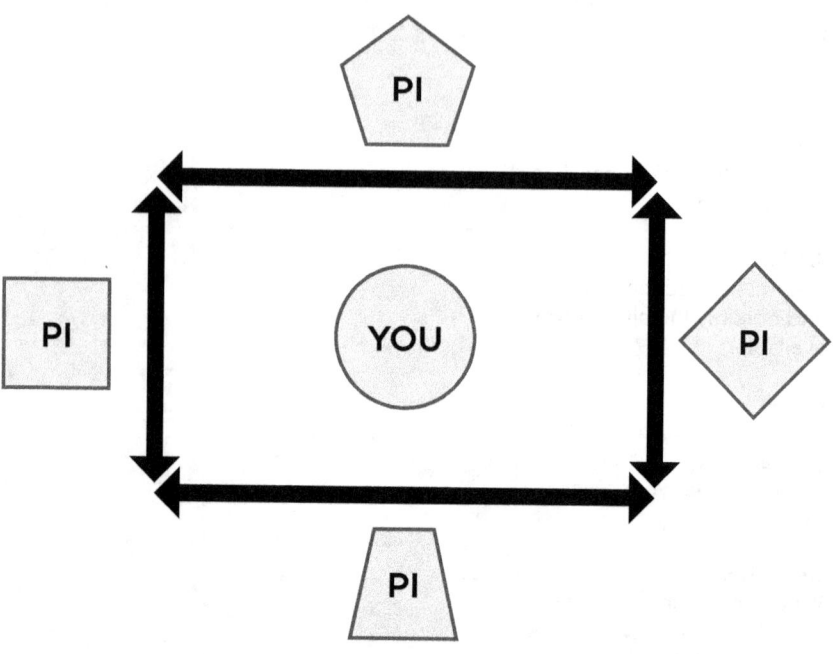

Do I have a trusting relationship with each of these individuals who may use their power of influence to support my success?

_____

_____

Does my organizational culture support diversity, equity, and inclusion (DEI)? If yes, what can be done from a systems level to improve the culture of DEI? If no, what can be done from a systems level to create a culture for DEI to thrive?

_____

_____

_____

_____

How do you use your power of influence to contribute to a culture of inclusive excellence?

2.4 → CODE-SWITCHING

1. Have you ever personally felt the need to "code-switch" or to "cover" an aspect of your identity? If yes, what were the circumstances?

2. How can your organization support your psychological safety in a way that empowers you to be your authentic self?

2.5 → IMPLICIT ASSOCIATION TEST

Complete the Harvard Implicit Association Test (IAT) to determine whether you have any biases toward any group(s). While your biases may be unconscious, they still have the potential to impact your relationships with others. You are encouraged to take the IAT multiple times involving different groups (https://implicit.harvard.edu/implicit/).

2.6 → FORMING A MENTOR RELATIONSHIP: ASSESS, IDENTIFY, REACH OUT

Assess
- Who do you consider a mentor?
- What attributes do you have in common?

Identify
- Identify two or three potential mentors.

Reach Out
- Ask to meet with a potential mentor to discuss the possibility of a formal mentoring relationship.

Assess: Has anyone invested in your career advancement that you would consider a mentor? What attributes did or do you have in common?

Identify: Are there any individuals in your organization or academic institution that you can identify as a potential mentor?

Reach out: If you have not reached out to this individual, establish a SMART goal for an initial meeting to discuss the possibility of a mentoring relationship.

REFERENCES

Alilyyani, B., Wong, C. A., & Cummings, G. (2018). Antecedents, mediators, and outcomes of authentic leadership in healthcare: A systematic review. *International Journal of Nursing Studies, 83*, 34–64. https://doi.org/10.1016/j.ijnurstu.2018.04.001

American Association of Colleges of Nursing. (2019). *Fact sheet: Enhancing diversity in the nursing workforce*. https://www.aacnnursing.org/News-Information/Fact-Sheets/Enhancing-Diversity

American Association of Colleges of Nursing. (2021). *The essentials: Core competencies for professional nursing education*. https://www.aacnnursing.org/Portals/42/AcademicNursing/pdf/Essentials-2021.pdf

American Nurses Association. (2020, September 11). New pulse on the nation's nurses survey series: COVID-19 pandemic financial impact greater for Black and Hispanic nurses. *Nursing World.* https://www.nursingworld.org/news/news-releases/2020/new-pulse-on-the-nations-nurses-survey-series-covid-19-pandemic-financial-impact-greater-for-black--and-hispaniclatino-nurses/

American Nurses Association. (2021, January 25). Leading nursing organizations launch the National Commission to Address Racism in Nursing. *Nursing World.* https://www.nursingworld.org/news/news-releases/2021/leading-nursing-organizations-launch-the-national-commission-to-address-racism-in-nursing/

Anderson, M. (2019, May 2). For black Americans, experiences of racial discrimination vary by education level, gender. *Pew Research Center.* https://www.pewresearch.org/fact-tank/2019/05/02/for-black-americans-experiences-of-racial-discrimination-vary-by-education-level-gender/

Beard, K. V., & Julion, W. A. (2016). Does race still matter in nursing? The narratives of African-American nursing faculty members. *Nursing Outlook, 64*(6), 583–596. https://doi.org/10.1016/j.outlook.2016.06.005

Beard, K. V., Julion, W., & Waite, R. (2020). Racism and the diversity policy paradox: Implications for nurse leaders. *Nursing Economic$, 38*(4), 176–178.

Bowen, D. J. (2020). Sponsoring diversity. *American College of Healthcare Executives blog.* https://www.ache.org/blog/2020/sponsoring-diversity

Cambridge Dictionary. (n.d.). *Authenticity.* https://dictionary.cambridge.org/us/dictionary/english/authenticity

Chakraborty, R. (2017). A short note on accent—Bias, social identity and ethnocentrism. *Advances in Language and Literary Studies, 8*(4), 57–64. http://dx.doi.org/10.7575/aiac.alls.v.8n.4p.57

Desai, S., Rao, S. A., & Jabeen, S. S. (2018, April 30). Developing cultural intelligence: Learning together with reciprocal mentoring. *Human Resource Management International Digest.* https://doi.org/10.1108/HRMID-03-2018-0050

Dunn, A. (2019, September 24). Younger college-educated black Americans are most likely to feel need to "code-switch." *Pew Research Center.* https://www.pewresearch.org/fact-tank/2019/09/24/younger-college-educated-black-americans-are-most-likely-to-feel-need-to-code-switch/

Earley, P. C., & Ang, S. (2003). *Cultural intelligence: Individual interactions across cultures.* Stanford University Press.

Eliades, A. B., Jakubik, L. D., Weese, M. M., & Huth, J. J. (2017). Mentoring practice and mentoring benefit 6: Equipping for leadership and leadership readiness—An overview and application to practice using mentoring activities. *Pediatric Nursing, 43*(1), 40–42.

Evans, J. D. (2013). Factors influencing recruitment and retention of nurse educators reported by current nurse faculty. *Journal of Professional Nursing, 29*(1), 11–20. https://doi.org/10.1016/j.profnurs.2012.04.012

Flanagin, A., Frey, T., Christiansen, S. L., & Bauchner, H. (2021). The reporting of race and ethnicity in medical and science journals: Comments invited. *JAMA, 325*(11), 1049–1052. https://doi.org/10.1001/jama.2021.2104

Fowler, B. A. (2020). Facilitators and barriers to leadership and career opportunities in minority nurses in public health departments. *Public Health Nursing, 37*(6), 821–828. https://doi.org/10.1111/phn.12800

Frazier, M. L., Fainshmidt, S., Klinger, R. L., Pezeshkan, A., & Vracheva, V. (2017). Psychological safety: A meta-analytic review and extension. *Personnel Psychology, 70*(1), 113–165. https://doi.org/10.1111/peps.12183

Fujimoto, Y., & Presbitero, A. (2021). Culturally intelligent supervisors: Inclusion, intercultural cooperation, and psychological safety. *Applied Psychology, 00*, 1–29. https://doi-org.proxy.lib.duke.edu/10.1111/apps.12326

Giles, H., & Coupland, N. (1991). *Language: Contexts and consequences*. Open University Press.

Godsil, R. D., Tropp, L. R., Goff, P. A., & Powell, J. A. (2014). Addressing implicit bias, racial anxiety, and stereotype threat in education and health care. *The Science of Equality, 1*, 1–90.

Goffman, E. (1963). *Stigma: Notes on the management of spoiled identity*. Prentice-Hall.

Guinaran, R. C., Alupias, E. B., & Gilson, L. (2021). The practice of power by regional managers in the implementation of an indigenous peoples health policy in the Philippines. *International Journal of Health Policy and Management, 10*, 402–413. https://doi.org/10.34172/ijhpm.2020.246

Iheduru-Anderson, K. (2020). Barriers to career advancement in the nursing profession: Perceptions of Black nurses in the United States. *Nursing Forum, 55*(4), 664–677. https://doi.org/10.1111/nuf.12483

Iheduru-Anderson, K., Shingles, R. R., & Akanegbu, C. (2021). Discourse of race and racism in nursing: An integrative review of literature. *Public Health Nursing, 38*, 115–130. https://doi.org/10.1111/phn.12828

Jakubik, L. D., Eliades, A. B., & Weese, M. M. (2016a). Part 1: An overview of mentoring practices and mentoring benefits. *Pediatric Nursing, 42*(1), 37–38.

Jakubik, L. D., Eliades, A. B., Weese, M. M., & Huth, J. J. (2016b). Mentoring practice and mentoring benefit 1: Welcoming and belonging—An overview and application to practice using mentoring activities. *Pediatric Nursing, 42*(2), 84–85.

Jakubik, L. D., Eliades, A. B., Weese, M. M., & Huth, J. J. (2016c). Mentoring practice and mentoring benefit 2: Mapping the future and career optimism—An overview and application to practice using mentoring activities. *Pediatric Nursing, 42*(3), 145–146.

Jakubik, L. D., Eliades, A. B., Weese, M. M., & Huth, J. J. (2016d). Mentoring practice and mentoring benefit 4: Supporting the transition and professional growth—An overview and application to practice using mentoring activities. *Pediatric Nursing, 42*(5), 252–253.

Jakubik, L. D., Eliades, A. B., Weese, M. M., & Huth, J. J. (2016e). Mentoring practice and mentoring benefit 5: Providing protection and security—An overview and application to practice using mentoring activities. *Pediatric Nursing, 42*(6), 300–301.

Jakubik, L. D., Weese, M. M., Eliades, A. B., & Huth, J. J. (2017). Mentoring in the career continuum of a nurse: Clarifying purpose and timing. *Pediatric Nursing, 43*(3), 149–152.

Johnson S. L. (2019). Authentic leadership theory and practical applications in nuclear medicine. *Journal of Nuclear Medicine Technology, 47*(3), 181–188. https://doi.org/10.2967/jnmt.118.222851

Livermore, D. (2011). *The cultural intelligence difference*. AMACOM.

Livermore, D. (2015). *Leading with cultural intelligence* (2nd ed.). AMACOM.

Livermore, D. (2016). *Driven by difference: How great companies fuel innovation through diversity*. AMACOM.

Matza, M. R., Garon, M. B., & Que Lahoo, J. (2018). Developing minority nurse leaders: The anchor and the rope. *Nursing Forum, 53*(3), 348–357. https://doi.org/10.1111/nuf.12261

McCluney, C. L., Robotham, K., Lee, S., Smith, R., & Durkee, M. (2019, November 15). The costs of code-switching. *Harvard Business Review*.

Moore, J. H., & Wang, Z. (2017). Mentoring top leadership promotes organizational innovativeness through psychological safety and is moderated by cognitive adaptability. *Frontiers in Psychology, 8*, 318.

Nardi, D., Waite, R., Nowak, M., Hatcher, B., Hines-Martin, V., & Stacciarini, J. M. R. (2020). Achieving health equity through eradicating structural racism in the United States: A call to action for nursing leadership. *Journal of Nursing Scholarship, 52*(6), 696–704. https://doi.org/10.1111/jnu.12602

National Academy of Medicine. (2021). *The future of nursing 2020–2030: Charting a path to achieve health equity*. The National Academies Press. https://doi.org/10.17226/25982

Rattan, A. (2021, June 10). Belonging in the workplace: Creating space for authentic self-expression. *Forbes*. https://www.forbes.com/sites/lbsbusinessstrategyreview/2021/06/10/belonging-in-the-workplace-creating-space-for-authentic-self-expression/?sh=2558f7556655

Shah, A. P. (2019). Why are certain accents judged the way they are? Decoding qualitative patterns of accent bias. *Advances in Language and Literary Studies, 10*(3), 128–139. https://doi.org/10.7575/aiac.alls.v.10n.3p.128

Simonsen, K. A., & Shim, R. S. (2019). Embracing diversity and inclusion in psychiatry leadership. *The Psychiatric Clinics of North America, 42*(3), 463–471. https://doi.org/10.1016/j.psc.2019.05.006

Smith, C. & Yoshino, K. (2019). Uncovering talent: A new model of inclusion [White paper]. *Deloitte.* https://www2.deloitte.com/content/dam/Deloitte/us/Documents/about-deloitte/us-about-deloitte-uncovering-talent-a-new-model-of-inclusion.pdf

Sullivan Commission. (2004). *Missing persons: Minorities in the health professions: A report of the Sullivan Commission on Diversity in the Healthcare Workforce.* https://campaignforaction.org/wp-content/uploads/2016/04/SullivanReport-Diversity-in-Healthcare-Workforce1.pdf

US Census Bureau. (2021). *Improved race and ethnicity measures reveal U.S. population is much more multiracial.* https://www.census.gov/library/stories/2021/08/improved-race-ethnicity-measures-reveal-united-states-population-much-more-multiracial.html

VeneKlasen, L., & Miller, V. (2002). Power and empowerment. *PLA Notes, 43*, 39–41.

Villarruel, A. M., & Broome, M. E. (2020). Beyond the naming: Institutional racism in nursing. *Nursing Outlook, 68*(4), 375–376. https://doi.org/10.1016/j.outlook.2020.06.009

Waite, R., & Nardi, D. (2017). Nursing colonialism in America: Implications for nursing leadership. *Journal of Professional Nursing, 35*(1), 18–25. https://doi.org/10.1016/j.profnurs.2017.12.013

Walter, A. W., Ruiz, Y., Tourse, R. W. C., Kress, H., Morningstar, B., MacArthur, B., & Daniels, A. (2017). Leadership matters: How hidden biases perpetuate institutional racism in organizations. *Human Service Organizations: Management, Leadership & Governance, 41*(3), 213–221. https://doi.org/10.1080/23303131.2016.1249584

Williams, D. R., Lawrence, J. A., & Davis, B. A. (2019). Racism and health: Evidence and needed research. *Annual Review of Public Health, 40*, 105–125. https://doi.org/10.1146/annurev-publhealth-040218-043750

Yoshino, K. (2006). *Covering: The hidden assault on our civil rights* (1st ed.). Random House.

"Knowing yourself is the beginning of all wisdom."
—**Aristotle, Greek philosopher**

3

Development and Application of Emotional Intelligence

The very essence of a crisis is that it is something outside of the norm that is straining the resources of typical functioning and adaptive coping. For the Covid-19 pandemic, while every person was in some way touched by fear, isolation, uncertainty, and financial insecurities, healthcare workers were called upon to directly work on the proverbial front lines and exposed to a debilitating and often lethal virus. In addition to the fear of contracting the virus, they were faced with moments of helplessness in not being able to heal their patients during Covid, regret over how quickly patients succumbed, frustration over the lack of adequate PPE supplies and politicization of public health measures to limit the transmission of the virus, and uncertainty about the future of

> **WE ASKED NURSE LEADERS**
>
> → How do you feel about what has happened?
>
> → What did you, your unit, and your hospital do to support staff during the Covid-19 crisis?

healthcare delivery. Further, many were faced with exhausting physical conditions in unwieldy protective gear, their noses and cheeks developing blisters from tight N95 masks, not to mention the mandatory overtime for some and the furloughs for others. Good leaders were not immune from facing the same physical, mental, and emotional challenges of their staff, often working side by side or even charging the way forward. In the middle of the "doing," however, was the very real need to feel and to process the emotions and the stress. During the interviews conducted with our leaders, one of the continual themes that emerged from all was the need for emotional intelligence to successfully handle their own stress and manage that of others.

EMOTIONAL INTELLIGENCE

Emotional intelligence (EI) is defined by the American Psychological Association (APA) Dictionary of Psychology as "a type of intelligence that involves the ability to process emotional information and use it in reasoning and other cognitive activities" (APA, n.d.). This concept of recognizing that specific knowledge, abilities, skills, and attitudes influence one's ability to cope and lead was first proposed in the mid-1960s by Michael Beldoch (1964) and then in a 1966 paper by B. Leuner. In 1990, psychologists Salovey and Mayer developed these constructs and proposed a framework for EI with four pillars, the ability to:

- Perceive and appraise emotions accurately

- Access and evoke emotions when they facilitate cognition

- Comprehend emotional language and make use of emotional information

- Regulate one's own and others' emotions to promote growth and well-being

Sometimes categorized as pop psychology, EI was quickly adopted with several different behavioral and psychological researchers proposing adaptation to different disciplines and refinements and debating definitions, terminology, and operationalization. Daniel J. Goleman is probably the most recognized for his writings on the topic, beginning with his first book, published in 1995, *Emotional Intelligence: Why It Can Matter More Than IQ*, and most recently, *The Emotionally Intelligent Leader* (2019).

GOLEMAN'S MODEL OF EMOTIONAL INTELLIGENCE

Goleman's evolving lens of EI as a mixed model with both ability and trait competencies as well as learned skills will be fully explored in this chapter. The model currently proposed by Goleman outlines five main EI constructs:

1. Self-awareness
2. Self-management
3. Motivation
4. Social awareness/skills
5. Empathy

Specific competencies within each domain aid in successful acquisition of EI. We found each of these concepts when interviewing our leaders and believe their experiences help to capture the essence of these constructs and modeling of leadership behaviors (Schwabel, 2011).

SELF-AWARENESS

Polonius, King Claudius' chief minister in Shakespeare's *Hamlet*, provides one of the most famous lines conceptualizing self-awareness: "To thine own self be true." Spoken to his son Laertes before his departure for university, Polonius provides blessings and guidance that have endured for over 500 years and are well worthy of republishing in this book of leadership principles. Take a minute to reflect on the passage in the nearby sidebar from Act 1, Scene 3.

POLONIUS TO LAERTES

Yet here, Laertes! Aboard, aboard, for shame!
The wind sits in the shoulder of your sail,
And you are stay'd for. There; my blessing with thee!
And these few precepts in thy memory
See thou character. Give thy thoughts no tongue,
Nor any unproportioned thought his act.
Be thou familiar, but by no means vulgar.
Those friends thou hast, and their adoption tried,
Grapple them to thy soul with hoops of steel;
But do not dull thy palm with entertainment
Of each new-hatch'd, unfledged comrade. Beware
Of entrance to a quarrel, but being in,
Bear't that the opposed may beware of thee.
Give every man thy ear, but few thy voice;
Take each man's censure, but reserve thy judgment.
Costly thy habit as thy purse can buy,
But not express'd in fancy; rich, not gaudy;
For the apparel oft proclaims the man,
And they in France of the best rank and station
Are of a most select and generous chief in that.
Neither a borrower nor a lender be;
For loan oft loses both itself and friend,
And borrowing dulls the edge of husbandry.
This above all: to thine ownself be true,
And it must follow, as the night the day,
Thou canst not then be false to any man.
Farewell: my blessing season this in thee!

Shakespeare, 2016

"Knowing thine self" means having emotional awareness, knowing both your strengths and weaknesses, drives, values, and goals. Self-awareness is allowing introspective prowess, self-confidence, and gut feelings to guide decisions.

We observed self-awareness in the nurse leaders we interviewed making choices about how much information they could emotionally handle related to Covid. Symone, our Education Coordinator for NICU, related:

"I had to make a decision that I was only going to deal with Covid for at least eight hours of my day. When I came home, I told my husband, it's fine if you want to watch [news programming], but can you watch it in another room? I couldn't deal with Covid all day at work and then come home and listen to the news because everything is contradicting anyway. I had to get real and be selective on how much I was going to let my brain absorb about this. And then I'd have to just check out or focus on decompressing to maintain my mental sanity. Working out, making sure I'm eating right, focusing on the kids. Trying your best to keep as normal of a life as you can around all this. And then start it all over tomorrow."

Symone, Education Coordinator for NICU

And Kathy, a Chief Nursing Officer for a Metro area hospital:

"I remember when I called [my husband], I got emotional at that point. Stuff within the hospital doesn't normally get me emotional. But I think the emotion came from, 'Oh my God, it's really happening. It's really here.' And we don't know what this is going to look like."

Kathy, Chief Nursing Officer

Another confirmed in a succinct manner:

> "I was very cognizant of how much I let into my head every day. I like to not get consumed with it."
>
> Vivian, Critical Care Unit Director

Self-awareness is not just having a firm grasp on our weaknesses or triggers, though; it is also having a firm awareness of what strengths or aspirations we bring to the table and the emotions that are driving us. Nancy recognized this when interacting with her staff, allowing herself to admit that she didn't have all the answers and didn't even understand how to personally process the mixture of overwhelming emotions and stress of the situation. For her, self-awareness allowed her to stop and process her emotions and be vulnerable and transparent with her colleagues:

> "So, I really had to do like a self-check, and how do I honestly feel about that? And I was just honest with the staff."
>
> Nancy, Critical Care Clinical Nurse Specialist

Overall, we found reluctance in the leaders to speak to their strengths. In our culture, perhaps that is due to a sense that to speak of strengths is to boast. However, when we combed through the interviews, we were able to find a few gems that our leaders did know what they were good at, supporting their role. Most of the time, these centered on stories of being good at developing relationships, of building trust, and of feeling a responsibility to lead the way in times of uncertainty as articulated by one leader:

> "Being able to have those relationships and able to have those conversations or having people I can have those conversations with is also a strength."
>
> Sharma, Director of Nursing Leadership

IMPROVING SELF-AWARENESS

There are numerous ways to develop your self-awareness skills, including:

- Paying attention to your thoughts and emotions
- Considering what bothers you about others and learning from example
- Developing a growth mindset
- Employing affirmative self-talk
- Journaling thoughts, plans, and actions
- Learning something new
- Limiting distractions and sources of negativity like social media
- Practicing meditation, prayer, or stillness
- Planning your activities and then evaluating your progress
- Reflecting on your experiences
- Seeking out constructive feedback
- Writing down your goals and aspirations

SELF-MANAGEMENT

The second domain of EI expression, self-management or self-regulation, involves controlling or redirecting emotions and impulses (both good and bad) and adapting to changing circumstances (Goleman, 2011). Building on self-awareness, self-management is successfully managing emotions and impulses appropriately to both maintain credibility and influence others. Nothing is perhaps as important in a crisis as when many turn to an effective leader who is "cool under fire." History has shown that the appointed leader is not always the one who emerges as the natural leader in crisis; instead, a crisis is often the critical juncture in which the ability (or not) to self-manage is revealed. Goleman proposed six necessary skills of leaders who are successful at self-management:

1. **Emotional self-control**: the ability to maintain effectiveness during difficult conditions and keep disruptive emotions and impulses in check.

2. **Transparency**: the ability to be clear and transparent with others about how you feel.

3. **Adaptability**: the flexibility to handle change, balance multiple demands, and adapt to new situations with fresh ideas.

4. **Achievement**: the ability to improve performance to meet personal standards.

5. **Taking initiative**: the ability to take action, demonstrate interest, and capitalize on opportunities.

6. **Optimism**: the ability to sustain hope and positive morale within an organization.

Self-management is the key behavioral component to self-awareness in this approach to authentic leadership. Self-management is the ability of a leader to draw upon and promote positive psychological capacities and a positive ethical climate through their composure and presence, thereby influencing calm and control (Northouse, 2016).

Sidney, a Nurse Manager at a Federally Qualified Health Center, reflected on two significant experiences that helped her overcome her fear of being exposed to Covid-19. The clinical nurse manager frequently referenced how overcoming her own fear allowed her to "lead by example" and mitigate the fear the nurses on her team might be experiencing as they conducted Covid-19 tests and cared for patients in the clinic:

"The very first thing—how I got over my fear, and it's the honest-to-God truth, two incidents happened. One, I actually got exposed to a person, and I had to take my temperature for 14 days and report my temperature every day. Since I was afebrile, I still came to work, but I had a mask on. This was in the beginning; that was the first. The second was when they asked me to go to the sick hotel—there's a hotel in Atlanta that's housing residents who were homeless but were positive for Covid. I was asked to go there and retrieve a urine specimen. It was unorthodox for me because that's not what we were doing; we weren't doing home visits then . . . and there was no process in place to do this, so I had to shoot from my hip, and I was [conflicted]."

Sidney, Federally Qualified Health Center Nursing Director

Her description of shooting from the hip and having to make a decision that was unprecedented based on her gut impulses was a clear example of self-awareness guiding self-management. She kept her emotions in check (emotional self-control) but was able to reflect on them as a moment of growth with transparency.

A component of EI, the necessity of adaptability in leadership during the pandemic has been unprecedented, so much so that Chapter 4 is devoted to adaptability and decision-making. But in the context of EI for purposes of completeness in this chapter, Nancy, our Critical Care Clinical Nurse Specialist, captured the need for adaptability, even in the face of the unknown, perfectly:

"In your mind, especially having medical training, and as a nurse, you're required to act. From the beginning, you're OK with acting quickly, you're OK with being in a crisis mode, and just adapting, going along with it, making the changes. I think you also recognize the authority, regulatory organizations so you are used to adapting."

Nancy, Critical Care Clinical Nurse Specialist

Having an achievement focus means that leaders envision and strive to make great things happen to achieve lofty objectives. An effective leader is able to identify an objective and gather the requisite expertise and passions of their individual team members to guide them in achieving high outcomes. The underlying motivation is superior performance. Achievement-oriented leaders are highly productive. One of our leaders discussed this achievement focus as a construct within self-management in the characteristics that distinguish a leader:

"A manager is someone who primarily guides and directs staff in tasks. The leader is able to look at what is being done, teach, support, provide feedback, analyze, and give more feedback. All done with encouragement and motivation, so that the people they are directing want to reach their goals. They are so motivating that the goal of the organization is now the employee's goal! Leaders to me are very charismatic. When they walk into the room, you want to hear what they have to say."

Nancy, Critical Care Clinical Nurse Specialist

Similarly, effective leaders don't wait to be told what to do. They take the initiative, finding and solving problems. Some may in fact accuse them of creating more work themselves as these types of leaders not only meet but create challenges. Highly self-managed or disciplined leaders find time to do more and feel a personal need to lead by example. Sometimes taking the initiative is looking at care from a new perspective and asking tough questions. One of the leaders we interviewed several times was Andrew, the Chief Quality Officer in Nursing for a large health system. When asked about how his team was monitoring quality with regards to Covid, he replied with the insight of an innovative leader:

"I will not say that we are doing anything new with regards to monitoring the quality of care for Covid patients specifically. But what we are doing is trying to figure out what the impact of all of these new processes, policies, procedures, how those may be impacting our quality measures. Let me give you an example. We have a system-level falls team initiative for the reduction of falls. And what we've noticed in the data is that we have had an increase in our fall rate since about the April time frame. What we're trying to do is figure that out, what's the reason for that—is it because we have patients who are a higher fall risk, or is it because we have a higher patient to staff ratio? Or what else goes into that fall rate? So . . . it's a matter of trying to figure out what the root causes of those things are. And if they are related to Covid, then developing some process to mitigate that specific thing."

Andrew, Chief Quality Officer in Nursing

> "What we're finding with falls is that the increased array tracks directly with our changes in our visitor policy, right? We can't have family at the bedside, and family is often more of a care partner than they are a visitor for our elderly or behavioral health or fall risk patients. So we think—and we haven't been able to prove it—but we think that the reduction in our visitors for patients because of Covid contributed to an increase in falls. So we're figuring out, how do we monitor or modify our visitor policy to get at least one person back in the room with the patient and see if that goes down? And if we do get the patients' families back in, and it [fall rates] doesn't go down, then we know that that wasn't the right thing, or we go some other direction. But it's really the same process as it always has been of taking each individual instance, trying to figure out what the cause of that instance was, and developing our charts to tell us which of the interventions we should tackle next."
>
> Andrew, Chief Quality Officer in Nursing

As the final component of self-regulation, optimism may have been thought to be lacking in our nurse leaders during the pandemic. But instead, what we heard time and again in our interviews was hope:

> "Yes, I'm sad [the pandemic is happening] because it's impacted so many lives. It's changed us—all of us—and how we interact with one another. Our work, our home, our social settings—it's just changed us in so many ways. So that part makes me a little sad, but then I am hopeful, because I do believe in possibility, and I believe that if we trust leaders who actually care about us, we can get through it."
>
> Andrew, Chief Quality Officer in Nursing

One of the most inspiring leaders we were able to interview was Amber, an Associate Professor, Psych-Mental Health Nurse Practitioner, and Nurse Entrepreneur who is well-regarded in the South for her multiple contributions to the health and welfare of children with cancer, pain, and psychological challenges. Her goal then and today is to create a sense of place where children can just be kids. What inspired us the most about Amber was her ability to stay focused on connecting and creating positive change. While she had a vision, it was her persistent energy and optimism that propelled a small endeavor with 40 children in the mid-1980s to becoming a multi-faceted system with ongoing programming throughout the year for children and their families. When Covid prevented children from attending programming, over 4,000 children benefited from "care in a box," scholarships, or Zoom teen nights. When asked about her personal feelings and challenges related to leading in the middle of Covid, she expressed not only optimism but each of the tenets of self-management:

"So yes, [the Covid crisis] really helped bring into focus what I realize are the most important things to me. [The crisis] hasn't changed anything. It's just sharpened it, and I'm grateful for that. I'm grateful that we're slowing down because I tend to be a person, both pre-Covid and it will be post-Covid, who is on the go . . . It energizes me and helps me be creative, and I really thrive on being with colleagues or patients, and that's when I feel like I do my best work. I think I've realized I can be effective and can do the things that I need to do remotely, though it may not be what I would choose to do. But it's helped me focus on what's the most important thing to me. And that is, again, connecting and creating positive change."

Amber, Nurse Entrepreneur and Associate Professor

> **IMPROVING SELF-MANAGEMENT**
> → Accept the emotion; control the response
> → Be mindful of your thoughts and feelings
> → Develop distress coping skills and tricks
> → Develop your communication skills
> → Know your emotional triggers
> → Own your response
> → Reframe challenges as opportunities
> → Set boundaries (know when to say no)
> → Step away physically or mentally for a few seconds if possible
> → When necessary, apologize

MOTIVATION

Those scoring high on internal motivation set high standards for themselves and others. These leaders are goal-driven, able to persist with attaining their goals, and intrinsically motivated. What drives them is the ability to never lose sight of the big picture, celebrate small milestones, and maintain the resiliency to power through.

Amber also discussed her own motivation and ability to stay optimistic during the pandemic, despite the temporary and frustrating delay in an objective she had devoted significant time and energy toward pre-Covid—the opening of a residential treatment facility for adolescents between 14–17 years of age:

"So, I think it's that safety first mindset . . . the thing that drives me, that motivates me with everything that I do? I'm thinking with the two organizations [that I developed and run], that it's those connections, that milieu, that community. Those are the important elements. How can we maintain them in this [Covid-19] environment safely?"

Amber, Nurse Entrepreneur and Associate Professor

HOW TO IMPROVE MOTIVATION
- → Create and repeat new positive habits
- → Develop small, measurable goals
- → Employ creativity
- → Focus on positivity
- → Limit extrinsic rewards
- → See and share the big picture
- → Simplify
- → Spread and celebrate results
- → Stay fueled
- → Take regular breaks
- → Utilize an accountability partner

SOCIAL AWARENESS AND EMPATHY

Having effective social skills as a leader consists of managing relationships in a way that benefits the organization. It is our ability to accurately identify the emotions of other people and understand what is motivating them. It means the leader must pay critical attention to the employee. Sit down. Stop talking. Look at the person and listen to what is being said. Instead of thinking about what should be said next, the authentic, socially aware leader listens and then formulates a response. By doing so, leaders will find they interrupt less and nonverbally impart that they value what the employee is saying.

Being socially aware is a critical skill. It allows the leader to "read the room" and gauge when discussions need to continue, when backtracking and allowing for understanding need to occur, and when consensus needs to be sought. Having excellent social skills for a leader means demonstrating proficiency in managing relationships and building networks, having the ability to find common ground and build rapport.

The need for social awareness during the pandemic was a point made by several nurse leaders as they described ensuring the frontline staff received food, time for self-care, encouragement to communicate with chaplains and the Faculty and Staff Assistance Program, and the need for regular feedback, praise, and celebration of successes. Leaders described regular rounding of units and taking the time to just sit and listen, to be available, and to remain positive. They intentionally worked on active listening and creating safe spaces for their staff.

Closely related to and difficult to dissect from social awareness is empathy. Defined as the ability to understand and appreciate another person's feelings and experiences (Oxford English Dictionary, 2021), it seems to us that empathy is more related to an understanding and feeling an emotional response to another's situation, whereas social awareness is the conscious acts or behaviors necessary to allow for the sharing of these emotions and development of empathy. As Brené Brown (2012, p. 81) relates: "Empathy has no script. There is no right way or wrong way to do it. It's simply listening, holding space, withholding judgment, emotionally connecting, and communicating that incredibly healing message of, 'You're not alone.'"

Similarly, our leaders discussed employing empathy:

"I have 14 people on my team, which for nursing leadership is a relatively small team. Having a small team, I think that I'm able to make more one-on-one connections with them and have more of a personal relationship. It's really hard to have a truly deep personal relationship with 100 people. But with my team, during Covid, that became even more important. Especially in the beginning, we just kind of sat around and talked about it. And I think that was . . . really needed during Covid."

Tanja, Unit Director for Labor and Delivery

"Ultimately, it is how we treat other human beings, whatever role you're in; it's that ability to connect and empathize and really understand and put yourself in the shoes of whoever's experiencing what."

Amber, Nurse Entrepreneur and Associate Professor

HOW TO IMPROVE SOCIAL AWARENESS
- Actively listen, focusing on what is said instead of what you will say next
- Call people by name; focus on remembering names
- Ask open-ended questions
- Compliment generously
- Employ icebreakers to start conversations
- Encourage others to talk about themselves
- Imitate others who are good at social skills
- Lean in as appropriate
- Make good eye contact
- Practice makes perfect
- Smile and remain confident
- Watch your body language

BUILDING EMPATHY
- Be culturally aware
- Be curious
- Be willing to share your own feelings
- Examine your biases
- Expand your knowledge with reading and culture
- Join in a shared cause
- Listen to other people
- Practice kindness intentionally
- Step out of your comfort zone
- Talk to new people
- Walk in the shoes of others

EMOTIONAL INTELLIGENCE IN NURSING

The development and enrichment of EI may be one of the most intentional approaches a nurse leader can directly employ. As described within this chapter, it is impossible to separate the emotional aspect of our beings from the workplace. We must acknowledge that those we care for, lead, and report to are all surrounded by individuals experiencing great highs and lows from births to deaths, recoveries to relapses, and successes to failures. Being able to readily recognize the emotions within oneself and others, use these emotions to reason, understand the emotions, and then manage them appropriately is what defines a highly emotionally intelligent nurse leader (Coladonato & Manning, 2017).

It has been proposed that EI is one of the professional skills that should be specifically developed in baccalaureate education as a means to improve academic success as well as well-being (Rankin, 2013), decrease student burnout, promote eventual compassion in the workplace, and decrease initial turnover rates once in practice. In addition, research directly correlates patient safety with EI by mediating the role of communication in patient safety and decreasing active system errors (Codier & Codier, 2015). Specific for nursing during the Covid-19 pandemic, a survey conducted in Tehran, Iran of nurses directly caring for patients with Covid-19 between May and July 2020 demonstrated just moderate scores of EI (Moradian et al., 2022). This suggests that these mentally and physically fatigued nurses could benefit from specific interventions focused on stabilizing and promoting resiliency (discussed in Chapters 9 and 10). Clearly, nurse leaders not only have a responsibility for developing their own EI but also modeling and developing it in their peers and team.

KEY TAKEAWAYS

Demonstrating EI is a cornerstone of effective leadership regardless of the exact model subscribed to. In our chapter, we reviewed Goleman's main constructs but clearly must acknowledge that these central themes are resonated in nearly every model. Some work emphasizes four pillars or shifts motivation under people skills, but the basic tenets and outcomes remain the same: Leaders who demonstrate EI are more apt to gain the trust of members of their team and increase productivity, morale, and retention of employees.

For an understanding of your level of EI, we recommend any number of leadership books on the topic but also taking a self-assessment test that can help identify areas that could be strengthened. Harvard Division of Continuing Education reviewed several of these self-assessments and recommend four at their website: https://professional.dce.harvard.edu/blog/assessing-your-emotional-intelligence-4-tools-we-love/

REFLECTIVE EXERCISES

3.1 → GOING WITH YOUR GUT

Describe a time when you had to make a decision or lead an initiative based on your gut instinct and self-confidence.

_____

_____

_____

_____

_____

_____

_____

3.2 → SELF-MANAGEMENT SKILLS ASSESSMENT

Based on analysis of the six necessary self-management skills, which has been the most challenging for you? What actions can you take to facilitate better integration into your leadership?

_____

_____

_____

_____

_____

_____

_____

3.3 → BREAKING DOWN A GOAL

Outside of a school or work responsibility, list a professional goal and break it into attainable subparts. For each step, determine what will keep you focused and help motivate actions to completion.

_____

_____

_____

_____

_____

_____

_____

3.4 → ACTIVE LISTENING

Describe a situation in which you felt your boss was actively listening to you. How did they make you feel heard? Describe their verbal and non-verbal communication. What about this situation will you borrow from in the future as a leader "hearing" a subordinate?

_____

_____

_____

_____

_____

_____

_____

3.5 → EMOTIONAL INTELLIGENCE ASSESSMENT

Take one of the self-assessments for EI listed on the Harvard website: https://professional.dce.harvard.edu/blog/assessing-your-emotional-intelligence-4-tools-we-love/. What insights did you gain? Are you surprised by the results? Identify one area for improvement and list three steps you can take to address it.

_____

_____

_____

_____

_____

_____

REFERENCES

American Psychological Association. (n.d.). *Emotional intelligence.* https://dictionary.apa.org/emotional-intelligence

Beldoch, M. (1964). Sensitivity to expression of emotional meaning in three modes of communication. In J. R. Davitz (Ed.), *The communication of emotional meaning* (pp. 31–42). McGraw-Hill.

Brown, B. (2012). Daring greatly: How the courage to be vulnerable transforms the way we live, love, parent, and lead. Gotham Books.

Codier, E., & Codier, D. (2015). A model for the role of emotional intelligence in patient safety. *Asia-Pacific Journal of Oncology Nursing, 2*(2), 112–117. https://doi.org/10.4103/2347-5625.157594

Coladonato, A. R., & Manning, M. L. (2017). Nurse leader emotional intelligence. *Nursing Management, 48*(9), 26–32. https://doi.org/10.1097/01.NUMA.0000522174.00393.f2

Goleman, D. (1995). *Emotional intelligence: Why it can matter more than IQ.* Bantam Books.

Goleman, D. (2011). *Leadership: The power of emotional intelligence.* More Than Sound.

Leuner, B. (1966). Emotional intelligence and emancipation. *Praxis der Kinderpsychologie und Kinderpsychiatrie, 15,* 193–203.

Moradian, S. T., Movahedi, M., Rad, M. G., & Saeid, Y. (2022). Emotional intelligence of nurses caring for COVID-19 patients: A cross-sectional study. *Archives of Psychiatric Nursing, 36,* 24–27. https://doi.org/10.1016/j.apnu.2021.10.011

Northouse, P. G. (2016). *Leadership: Theory and practice* (7th ed.). Sage Publications.

Oxford English Dictionary. (2021). In *Oxford English dictionary online.* https://www-oed-com.

Rankin, B. (2013). Emotional intelligence: Enhancing value-based practice and compassionate care in nursing. *Journal of Advanced Nursing, 69*(12), 2717–2725.

Salovey, P., & Mayer, J. D. (1990). Emotional intelligence. *Imagination, Cognition and Personality, 9*(3), 185–211. https://doi.org/10.2190/DUGG-P24E-52WK-6CDG

Schawbel, D. (2011, September 15). Daniel Goleman on leadership and the power of emotional intelligence. *Forbes.* https://www.forbes.com/sites/danschawbel/2011/09/15/daniel-goleman-on-leadership-and-the-power-of-emotional-intelligence/?sh=561adfce6d2f

Shakespeare, W. (2016). Hamlet. In B. Mowat & P. Werstine (Eds.), *The Folger Shakespeare library* (Original work published 1599). https://www.folgerdigitaltexts.org/html/Ham.html#line-1.3.0

> *"The most important factor for survival is neither intelligence nor strength but adaptability."*
> —**Charles Darwin, British naturalist**

4

Adaptability and Decision-Making

All living creatures are forced to adapt to survive. For humankind, these adaptations may be conscious or unconscious, successful or unsuccessful, filled with ease with the hope of opportunity or mired in conflict, anxiety, and fear. Certainly, the pandemic has forced on all of humankind certain adaptations for how we educate, work, deliver healthcare, worship, and socialize. New terms such as "social distancing" have been coined and new norms formed such as distance learning, Zoom meetings, and telehealth appointments.

Every organization has been affected by the pandemic, but the healthcare system faced unprecedented challenges. Foremost was the

---

WE ASKED NURSE LEADERS

→ What sources, data, and information did you use to determine changes in policies and procedures?

→ How did you handle new revelations or guidelines about treating the virus?

→ What did you rely on to help guide your actions as you had to adapt?

need to deliver care that was effective. In the early weeks and months, unsure of effective treatment strategies and perhaps complicated by patients arriving too late to the hospital, early case fatality rates topped 6.25% in May of 2020 (compared to rates less than 1.6% at the end of 2021; Ritchie et al., 2022).

During this same period, frontline staff were not clear on the transmissibility and how to stay safe. There were shortages of PPE supplies and critical equipment like ventilators, cleaning products, hand sanitizer, and paper products. Multiple unknowns complicated care, like how to perform CPR while limiting spread of the virus, if new mothers infected with the virus should nurse their newborns, if masks could be sterilized and reused, how long it took to turn over a room from an infected person, etc. When one problem was addressed, another popped up, often related to an attempt to solve the first. These stressful conditions forced everyone in healthcare to adapt to "new norms" while attempting to balance fears and ever-changing information. Leadership during such tumultuous times requires extreme agility and can be likened to an ever-changing combat situation. Core to this stress is that decisions must be made, sometimes so many at one time that those in leadership become overwhelmed.

ADAPTIVE LEADERSHIP

One strategy proposed for leadership during situations such as this is adaptive leadership. First articulated by Heifetz et al. in 2009, this model of leadership draws on the concept of evolutionary biology to mobilize people and resources to tackle tough challenges and thrive. Adaptive leadership is not necessary in all situations but is useful during times of crisis.

Specifically hailing from adaptive evolution, the concept of thriving asserts that changes in the environment allow the organism to adapt to its habitat. Adaptive leadership is facilitating change not through providing known solutions but refashioning people's priorities, beliefs, habits, and loyalties. Adaptive leaders do not have all the expert knowledge to impart the correct response to the environmental threats; rather, they mobilize experts and other resources to allow for discovery and experimentation, celebrating even small successes and generating capacity to thrive anew.

Adaptive leadership must be differentiated from the routine leadership provided in the average day. As defined by Sharon Daloz Parks (2005), routine leadership deals with technical problems that may be complex but can be solved with knowledge and procedures already in place. Adaptive challenges require new learning, innovation, and new patterns of behavior.

The original principles of adaptive leadership (Heifetz et al., 2009) are outlined below. During the middle of a crisis when decisions must be made and answers provided, these five components can help with quickly assessing the situation, seeking appropriate input, attempting a solution, and then constantly evaluating the results and supporting the staff. These key components were often found in the interviews with our leaders:

- **Build on the past:** Adaptive leaders successfully adapt by making the best possible use of prior knowledge, insights, and experiences.

- **Experiment:** Adaptation involves being open to innovation, improvisation, and then critical evaluation of effectiveness.

- **Rely on diversity:** Adaptive leaders build a culture that values diverse views and relies on the strength of various perspectives.

- **Re-regulate:** Change causes disarray and requires re-regulation or modification to filter the most important information and to address it.

- **Persistence:** Adaptation takes time. Therefore, adaptive leadership requires persistence or a continued course of action in spite of difficulty or opposition (Oxford English Dictionary, 2021).

The following are some excerpts from the interviews conducted with the leadership mentors that speak to each of the five adaptive leadership principles.

BUILDING ON THE PAST

One of the basic tenets of healthcare leadership is preparation through policies, procedures, and drills for disasters. The Joint Commission has included emergency preparedness in its regulations since 1995, first as a component of the Environment of Care section and then expanding into its own independent chapter in 2009 following significant disasters across the country that overwhelmed healthcare resources. These included terroristic mass casualty events in the World Trade Center attacks, global power outages, and weather-related events (hurricanes and tornados). Fears had been mounting for about a decade when President Obama called on members of Congress to put aside partisan politics to pass funding necessary to combat pandemics in the future, in 2014:

> "There may and likely will come a time in which we have both an airborne disease that is deadly, and in order for us to deal with that effectively we have to put in place an infrastructure, not just here at home but globally, that allows us to see it quickly, isolate it quickly, respond to it quickly, so that if and when a new strain of flu like the Spanish flu crops up five years from now or a decade from now, we've made the investment and we're further along to be able to catch it."
>
> **–Barack Obama, former President**

However, the funding was not approved.

Key to preparedness is a thorough understanding of our present and past. Well-engrained into the mission of the Centers for Disease Control and Prevention (CDC, 2022, para. 3) is a pledge to "base all public health decisions on the highest quality scientific data that is derived openly and objectively."

This data is our past: how many, with what lethality, what worked, what failed, what was the cause? The adaptive leadership approach proposed by the Heifetz Model is focused on an epidemiological perspective that values lessons learned, utilizing them to prevent, treat, and mitigate.

Effective adaptable leadership of an organization, even a healthcare organization struggling to contain a pandemic, builds on the past. Several leaders shared stories of past emergency preparedness measures and activation of plans for small and large events. From each of these situations, thoughtful evaluation resulted in plan revision or updated protocols, creating an iterative process of refinement.

Building on the past encompasses building on the evidence. Kimberly, Nurse Anesthetist and Nursing Faculty, discussed basing decisions and plans on key concepts of Maslow's Hierarchy for provision of safety:

> "As long as people are afraid for their lives, so to speak, they're afraid they're going to get this virus…they do not feel safe. We have to meet lower-level needs of food, shelter, and safety. Until those are met, you're not going to be able to function at a higher level and deliver care to a patient."
>
> Kimberly, Nurse Anesthetist and Nursing Faculty

However, drawing from past knowledge and experience doesn't always prepare us completely. "We had a policy that covered everything in terms of disaster, and it did mention pandemic. But…" This manager went on to list how it provided a good start but was incomplete because the situation entered into with Covid-19 was not what was anticipated years prior when the policy had been developed.

Carson, Vice President of Nursing Practice and Education, described feeling well-positioned for effective management of Covid patients since they had cared for persons with Ebola:

"During the West Africa Ebola outbreak, we treated a handful, maybe four or five Ebola patients that were very sick, and they survived. We also treated other people that had been exposed to Ebola and monitored but who never got sick. So, to that extent there, we had some experience of a limited few people with a deadly, highly contagious pathogen. And I think early on, we thought because of our Ebola work, we were like, 'OK, we're ready for this.' But we learned very quickly that Covid was a whole different beast."

Carson, Vice President of Nursing Practice and Education

He went on to describe how safely being able to care for persons with Ebola helped to inform some of the initial response. But the organization and their adaptive leaders were forced to try new strategies and experiment when the necessary response had never been attempted in the past.

EXPERIMENTATION

From an organizational perspective, those seeking to lead adaptive change need an experimental mindset. They must learn to improvise as they go, both creating and implementing several different tactics to achieve specified objectives. By pursuing several approaches, the adaptive leader is able to better identify strategies for the next level of change, yielding results that improve with each step. During a crisis, multiple needs demand solutions at once. Necessity is the driver of innovation, and healthcare systems around the country rose to the occasion through experimentation with solutions to problems of PPE and staff shortages, novel and investigational treatments, and even staff onboarding and orientation. While far from a complete list, issues verbalized by the interviewed leaders requiring experimentation to balance effective care for patients while assuring health workers, safety included:

- Testing, tracking, and informing patients and staff of Covid status
- Deploying nurses outside of their comfort zone and avoiding furloughs
- Providing necessary orientation, education, and training in some instances while deferring in others
- Vetting and prioritizing need for surgical procedures
- Communicating critical information via new methods
- Assuring compliance with HIPAA standards while imparting necessary information to ensure staff, patient, and family safety
- Setting up specialty Covid units to allow for cohorting of patients
- Meeting isolation needs in the face of PPE shortage
- Implementing clinical trials with new medications
- Collaborating and team building in an entirely new way
- Restricting visitation, necessitating revision of communication approaches with family and loss of the personal care and attendance families provided
- Implementing new means of healthcare delivery such as telehealth
- Safely delivering risky interventions such as general anesthesia, CPR, and intubation via means to prevent aerosolization of virus to staff

When asked about experimenting with different solutions, the leaders we interviewed were virtual founts, overflowing with the multitude of changes they had helped facilitate or devised:

> "We get into some really cool things! I mean, we challenged the hospital standard!"
>
> Michelle, Innovation and Advancement Coordinator

> "Our Education Coordinator had to really look at what was absolutely necessary and what could be done online, what could be distributed. We took that two-day down to a one-day orientation. Then we had to help these nurses that were being redeployed be comfortable in other settings. So we took their med/surg orientation and omitted sections to limit it to four hours with essential information for nursing."
>
> Rebecca, Director of Nursing Education

> "We still need to onboard people. We definitely need nurses throughout this. I love the fact that we are utilizing Zoom for everything."
>
> Symone, Education Coordinator for NICU

> "So many different things: limiting the number of staff in breakrooms at one time. Mandating masks at all times in each unit. Different formats for posting meetings because Covid is here, but life still has to go on. So, we still need to meet, we still need to teach, we still need to educate and all that good stuff."
>
> Jane, Nurse Practitioner Ambulatory Care

> "We'll start out in one direction and they can change directions at any time, and when it does, you have to be ready for the change. We know that this is a growing process especially with the pandemic."
>
> Andrew, Chief Quality Officer in Nursing

Foundational to this crisis was that many, if not all, healthcare facilities across the country and the world were facing the same crises and struggling with the same issues. A multitude of solutions have emerged, been shared, and published. To close the loop with adaptive experimentation, these results should be analyzed and compared so that best practices can be identified, fleshed out into policies proactive of future crises, and further experimentation undertaken.

VALUING DIVERSITY

For organizations, adaptive leadership recognizes that those usually in charge may not have all the answers. In television dramas, when there is a problem, we see the classic brainstorming of ideas around a conference table with the wildest strategy proposed by the youngest partner just in time to save the day. But valuing the ideas and ingenuity of others is a long-standing precept of successful leaders from Confucius to Jack Welch and Ronald Reagan. Each is reported to have some quote that centers on the need to surround themselves with people smarter than themselves in order to attain success. This central construct of adaptive leading is to rely less on central planning and the genius of the few at the top and more on the ingenuity of others with diverse education, viewpoints, and positions.

In non-crisis times, leaders typically turn to the evidence and authorities for direction, and clearly the CDC and World Health Organization provided significant guidance at every stage of this pandemic. But having no research or previous experience with this coronavirus, even the experts were required to engage stakeholders to make consensus decisions and borrow from similar situations with hopes that the same approach would work. For many of these dilemmas, this approach worked, yet at other times, high-profile decisions or suggestions were put forth but then later had to be amended, or even retracted.

Successful adaptive leaders reported valuing multiple opinions in trying to make the best decision. They reported consulting with scientists, others around the country, and those on the front lines delivering the care. Amber, Nurse Entrepreneur and Professor, described her approach to assembling her team at the beginning of the pandemic:

"This is a reality; I'm going to do this, we're going to do this; here's this gap and here's my goal. I had a timeline, I had some structure to it, but it's pulling those folks together to get their expertise and being receptive and open. That is magical."

Amber, Nurse Entrepreneur and Associate Professor

Adaptive leaders assemble the right people at the table and identify the problem. They view the situation as an opportunity and entertain suggested solutions:

"In your mind, especially having medical training, and as a nurse, you're required to act. From the beginning, you're OK with acting quickly, you're OK with being in a crisis mode, and just adapting, going along with it, making the changes. I think you also recognize the authority, regulatory organizations, so you are used to adapting. Next comes acceptance. And that is where you see this has a complexity and a duration that is challenging you to think differently in every area that you haven't before. You then start to see it as opportunity. A big part of the opportunity is relying on other people. You're reaching out for solutions to solve problems and really working together to bring in other perspectives."

Nancy, Critical Care Clinical Nurse Specialist

"I would raise my hand, as well as others who would raise their hand, and say, give a try, take it on or just step in and say, 'I know a little bit about that. I can take that on.' It really wasn't necessarily based on anyone's expertise; it was based on our willingness to reach out to people who we thought could help drive requirements and process the policy, and then quickly lead a team to do it."

Andrew, Chief Quality Officer in Nursing

RE-REGULATION

Learning is often painful. New adaptations often lead to feelings of being displaced, feeling incompetent, betrayed, or irrelevant. Not many people like to be "rearranged." Leadership therefore requires the diagnostic ability to recognize those losses and the predictable defensive patterns of response that operate at the individual and systemic level. An adaptive leader recognizes these responses in employees and takes steps to prevent, address, and mitigate them. Several of our leaders spoke to helping their employees re-regulate, like Rebecca, Director of Nursing Education, who recognized the challenges of being deployed to new areas:

"It is stressful to be redeployed. If you are working in ambulatory all of the time and then have to go back to inpatient, it's a big switch, and I realize that we really have to support those nurses. That is when we realized that this is going to be a little bigger than we initially thought."

Rebecca, Director of Nursing Education

And Kimberly (Nurse Anesthetist and Nursing Faculty), who said:

"One area where we have seen a lot of people struggle to adapt to is in mask compliance. To me, it was really interesting to see how challenging and difficult that was, for people who work in healthcare to accept this and just wear a mask."

Kimberly, Nurse Anesthetist and Nursing Faculty

Direct training was limited to skills the redeployed nurse felt comfortable with, and creating nursing care teams accompanied nurse redeployment. Instead of a floating nurse taking a full patient assignment, they were paired with a unit nurse who oversaw all aspects of critical care while the redeployed nurse was assigned tasks well within their wheelhouse. The redeployed nurses were supported at every step in the process and valued for the touch and time they brought to a critical situation; they were celebrated just as the heroes providing more critical, life-sustaining care.

At times, there was a need to help patients adapt to something they felt was pejorative:

"We've had a couple of patients that were definitely like, 'This is a hoax; it's created by 5G,' etc. Unfortunately, one of those patients was symptomatic, so that was a challenge. She wouldn't be tested, and then she was very angry that we were coming into her room in full PPE. And she didn't want to keep her mask on."

Tanja, Unit Director Labor and Delivery

Tanja went on to relate how framing this conversation with the patient was the most significant:

> "That was the most challenging situation where we actually had to initiate a behavioral contract, which we do sometimes with patients, that basically says, 'These are the expectations that we need you to follow if we're going to continue to provide you care here in the hospital.' It outlines what you need to do, and one of those things is, 'You don't have to believe in Covid, but you have to wear a mask when we're in your room.' We had to adopt a team approach with nursing leadership, the patient's nurse, the physician, and security. And so we all had to gown up and go in and have that conversation with her. And it worked! I mean, it usually does when they see that everybody's on the same page."
>
> Tanja, Unit Director Labor and Delivery

PERSISTENCE

Probably the easiest pillar to understand is that adaptive leadership requires persistence and takes time. Significant change is the product of incremental experiments that build over time. Leaders discussed time and again just putting one foot in front of another and persisting. Trying something new, letting other things go. And waking up to realize six months had passed, valuing how far they had come, and marveling at the work accomplished:

"Yes, it's been crazy. If we look back now, it's hard to believe it. In some ways, it's hard to believe it's been six months. And then in other ways, it's hard to even remember what things were like before all this started."

Jane, Nurse Practitioner Ambulatory Care

But persistence alone is not the answer to managing the situation when time is of the essence. As related by Andrew, Chief Quality Officer in Nursing, before persistence is prioritization:

"Everything was, we need it done yesterday. But that's just about time, dedication, right? A lot of times in normal work, we don't necessarily prioritize very well. I'll jump from one task to another task. But in that situation, we had to just prioritize, and we had to kind of take things one at a time."

Andrew, Chief Quality Officer in Nursing

Finally, there comes a point when the adaptive leader recognizes that the situation will never return to a pre-crisis state. We will all talk of pre-pandemic days, or how healthcare used to be, while fully recognizing that some practices will never be the same. Irrevocably changed. And that with persistence comes acceptance and resolution.

"I think we've realized that this is going to be with us for a long time, and we just need some more sustainable practices on how we're going to move forward because it's not going away. There's a huge difference between where we were at when we started and where we're at now . . . At the beginning, we didn't really know anything. So hopefully, we'll continue to move forward."

Tanja, Unit Director Labor and Delivery

REMODELING ADAPTIVE LEADERSHIP

The adaptive leadership theory by Heifetz and colleagues was originally put forth as a marketing model where experimentation could lead to temporary losses of money or market share that, in business risk decisions, can be acceptable. Part of the beauty of this model was that this experimentation, with known possible losses, was encouraged because with experimentation and employment of three or more different approaches to a campaign, direct head-to-head comparison could be made and a clear winner identified. The successful campaign or tactic would hopefully negate the approaches that lost money, or in some instances, could continue with justification that they appealed to a certain smaller segment of the population while the more lucrative approach appealed to a more mainstream crowd.

It is one thing to have acceptable losses in advertising, but losses within healthcare and the military are quite another. Michael Useem (2010), Professor of Management and Director of the Center for Leadership and Change at the Wharton School at the University of Pennsylvania, values some additional key approaches in teaching adaptive leadership from a military lens, where losses are not acceptable and must be minimized. Building on several of the key tenets, he suggests that a military leader employs four additional tactics of adaptive leadership that can be directly employed during a military crisis. Dr. Rose Sherman (2014) suggested that these leadership tactics may be useful in healthcare crises in her blog, books, and various speaking engagements concerning nursing leadership:

- Be present
- Make decisions
- Focus on the mission
- Convey strategic intent

BE PRESENT

Foremost is to be present with those on the front lines. This principle creates personal links with those being led through challenging times by showing up, taking time to personally interact, encourage, and hear subordinates. While this is sometimes difficult because there are so many shifting priorities and meetings, staff must see those in command, feel valued, and feel engaged. Our leaders recognized quickly that while an issue with direct patient care may have bubbled up to the director level, it is absolutely critical that the bedside clinical nurses be involved with developing the solution. Further, especially during such times of crisis, nurse leaders are key to helping re-arranged staff re-regulate and adapt. Our leaders spoke several times of offering this support to their clinical nurses:

> "So for me, my main concern was to make sure the staff was OK, [by] rounding on them, checking on them, following up, making sure they have what they need, making sure that, although we're in the middle of a crisis, we are actually recommending taking time for self-care, which is very difficult to do . . . to be out there in the front line and caring for the patient. I wanted to make sure that they were OK. I wanted to make sure that they had meals. That they were part of the program that had meals delivered to them. That we've partnered with our chaplains to offer some perks for them even while at work, so they can have some sort of self-care moments as well."
>
> Vivian, Critical Care Unit Director

MAKE DECISIONS

Hand in hand with experimentation is the requisite to make decisions. While it may not be the perfect call, the adaptive leader must make good and timely decisions. Useem suggests adopting the Marine dictum that when you are 70% ready and have 70% agreement, then act (2010). Use the information, evidence, and intuition you have at that time to make the best decision possible. Directly related to this is recognizing that the leader's responsibility is to make the best decision at the time and then re-evaluate. Leaders (and their staff) must accept that the perfect decision will not be made every time, but sometimes the only way to recognize that you are on the wrong trail is to start down it and evaluate. You may have to turn around and you may have to blaze a way through the underbrush to get on the right path, but the journey has been started and progress made.

Decision-making can be elaborated on by examining the tenets used by those in public health. A key point is that the quality of a decision—in this case, for crisis decision-making—cannot be judged by the outcome. A good decision can have a bad outcome, and a bad decision can have a good outcome (Hammond et al., 2002; Howard & Abbas, 2015; Spetzler et al., 2016). Decisions are based on reasoning, both causal and probabilistic. Causal reasoning addresses the root causes, the key drivers, why and how is this happening, how the countermeasures are evaluated, and if they will be effective in the real world. Probabilistic reasoning is much more difficult to address as it is based on prediction and conjecture (e.g., "What are the chances . . . ?").

The pandemic presented a level of uncertainty on a massive scale, clearly magnifying the difficulty in decision-making. The dimensions of such uncertainty can be defined by what can be known and what is known. In trying to ascertain what is known, the following questions are asked (Aragón et al., 2021):

1. The *known knowns:* What do we know that we know? Use it.
2. The *known unknowns:* What do we know that we don't know? Assemble it (i.e., the information is available to us).

3. The *unknown knowns:* What do we not know that others know? Seek it (e.g., information that is hidden from us, including blind spots).

4. The *unknown unknowns:* What do we not know that others don't know either? Imagine it (e.g., "what if" scenario planning).

From that initial decision and those first steps, processes develop that can be further refined as discussed here with Andrew, Chief Quality Officer in Nursing, who had to develop an approach for the early dissemination of Covid test results:

"Probably the very first thing that I worked on was trying to figure out how to get Covid results back to patients. Myself and our epidemiology laboratory director sat and called patients for about three hours. That's not something that I typically do, but she would call the positives, I would call the negatives, and then we'd put a note in the chart. So just trying to adapt to the needs at the moment and then from there, we grew processes for manning the patient call centers, for scheduling Covid testing, and managing and communicating results. Everything kind of grew out of those initial days, when we were all just kind of scrambling and going: 'OK, how do we do this?' We've got to make something happen within the next hour, the next day. Trying to make a huge ship that typically takes weeks or months to make something happen overnight."

Andrew, Chief Quality Officer in Nursing

FOCUS ON THE MISSION

Focusing on the mission is the third tactic in which the leader must establish a common purpose with those being led. Every coach and military commander knows this tactic and employs it readily to focus the team on a unified objective. Sharing a common purpose is a cornerstone to tackling difficult situations, overcoming obstacles, and creating allies. Redeployment of staff was a challenging task that Andrew discussed having to set up using key input from critical partners. He describes assembling the right stakeholders and experts and laying out their objective:

"I co-led the staff redeployment effort with our HR staff, our HR lead, and our staffing pool lead. That was building an office from nothing, it was building a staff redeployment office . . . We also went through that effort that I talked about—the critical care team model. I led that with the Director of Professional Development. I used to be a critical care nurse; I'm not anymore but I have some background in that area. We basically pulled in a bunch of critical care clinical nurse specialists and critical care nurses to say: 'OK, here's the goal. Our goal is to figure out how to take care of critical care patients when we don't have enough nurses to do it. And what are options to do that?'"

Andrew, Chief Quality Officer in Nursing

CONVEY STRATEGIC INTENT

Closely related with focusing on the mission is to convey strategic intent: Make the objectives clear but allow those who will be executing the actions to determine the best approach and procedures. Usually, those closest to the situation are best able to operationalize the goal. Amber, our Nurse Entrepreneur and Professor, recognized this, assuring that those who would be delivering care and interacting with clients were involved in the decisions regarding these interactions:

"We're all at the table. Yes, we know what our goal is. I obviously had structure in mind and pieces of it, but just to utilize that, the talent and passion of the team to really fill in those gaps and put the additional substance to that program, and watching that, and being a part of it, but it's not at my directive, it's taking that time to pull that group together. So that together you can create!"

Amber, Nurse Entrepreneur and Associate Professor

KEY TAKEAWAYS

According to Coccia (2020), management of critical decisions is the process by which an organization deals with a disruptive and unexpected event that threatens to harm the organization or its stakeholders. Typically, the disruptive situation presents (a) as a threat to the organization, (b) with an element of surprise, and (c) requires critical decisions to be made in a short amount of time.

Our interviews with various leaders of healthcare organizations during the first year of the Covid pandemic revealed the challenges of having to adapt and make critical decisions on every level of care as pandemic supplies, testing, vaccinations, and treatments evolved. The enormity of the decisions, often that involved life and death, coupled with the time-sensitivity and a fair margin of politics were experienced by all:

"You know, it's kind of an all-hands-on-deck situation. It was a mix of being willing and being capable of taking on a team and putting them through a formal approach to assessing a problem, collaborating on what potential solutions could be, and then defining our options to the leadership team and making the final decision."

Symone, Education Coordinator for NICU

"We had to figure out what the scope of those things were too; what were the deadlines around doing it and how critical were they? What was the scope of what we were supposed to do versus what was out of bounds for us to do? Plus, we had to work quickly, like in the Intermediate Care Unit, our job was to define what the criteria guidelines trigger points and process are for setting up an Immediate Care Unit."

Andrew, Chief Quality Officer in Nursing

Adaptive leadership provides a framework for facing a crisis and making critical decisions. Nurse leaders clearly demonstrated the skill set to identify and adapt to the multiple challenges at hand and to make decisions under extremely difficult situations. In the next chapter, we will look at the creative ways they addressed the areas identified for change.

REFLECTIVE EXERCISES

4.1 → TECHNICAL AND ADAPTIVE CHALLENGES

Based on your understanding of technical problems as opposed to adaptive challenges, make a list of the types of issues you were faced with prior to the pandemic. In the column to the right, identify whether this would be a technical or adaptive challenge encountered during the pandemic.

Challenge	Technical or Adaptive

Challenge	Technical or Adaptive

4.2 → ADDRESSING AN ADAPTIVE CHALLENGE

Choose one challenge from the list you created in Exercise 4.1. Identify key principles of adaptive leadership that would help you address the situation. List strategies, identifying necessary people, implementation strategies, and how the effectiveness would be evaluated.

Challenge

Strategy

Necessary People

Implementation

Evaluation Methods

4.3 → EVALUATING STRATEGIES

Think back to early days and later days of the pandemic and identify strategies presented by Useem that were employed by leaders you worked with or for. What strategies made you feel valued and committed? Did these continue as the pandemic stretched resources and patience over the past two years, or were some dropped?

Early Strategies

Later Strategies

4.4 → AREA OF IMPROVEMENT

Using the STARR technique, describe a specific decision required during the pandemic. Then identify the tasks involved, what actions you took, the result of those actions, and what you might do differently in the future.

Situation Describe the challenging situation.	
Task Describe the task at hand or target desired.	
Action Describe the actions taken and possibly the alternatives available.	

Result Describe the outcome of your actions, including the ability to meet your objective.	
Reflection What did you learn? What would you do differently, the same, or better next time being posed with a similar situation?	

REFERENCES

Aragón, T., Cody, S., Farnitano, C., Hernandez, L., Morrow, S. A., Pan, E. S., Tzvieli, O., & Willis, M. (2021). Crisis decision-making at the speed of COVID-19: Field report on issuing the first regional shelter-in-place orders in the United States. *Journal of Public Health Management and Practice, 27*, S19–S28. https://doi.org/10.1097/PHH.0000000000001292

Centers for Disease Control and Prevention. (2022). *Pledge to the American people.* https://www.cdc.gov/about/organization/pledge.html

Coccia, M. (2020). Critical decision in crisis management: Rational strategies of decision making. *Journal of Economics Library, 7*(2), 81–96.

Hammond, J. S., Keeney, R. L., & Raiffa, H. (2002). *Smart choices: A practical guide to making better decisions.* Crown Business.

Heifetz, R., Grashow, A., & Linsky, M. (2009). *The practice of adaptive leadership: Tools and tactics for changing your organization and the world.* Harvard Business Press.

Howard, R. A., & Abbas, A. E. (2015). *Foundations of decision analysis* (1st ed.). Pearson.

Obama, B. (2014). Remarks at the National Institutes of Health in Bethesda, Maryland. *The American Presidency Project.* https://www.presidency.ucsb.edu/node/308005

Oxford English Dictionary. (2021). https://www.oed.com

Parks, S. D. (2005). *Leadership can be taught: A bold approach for a complex world*. Harvard Business School.

Ritchie, H., Mathieu, E., Rodés-Guirao, L., Appel, C., Giattino, C., Ortiz-Ospina, E., Hasell, J., Macdonald, B., Beltekian, D., & Roser, M. (2022). *Coronavirus pandemic (COVID-19)*. https://ourworldindata.org/coronavirus

Sherman, R. O. (2014). *Adaptive leadership*. https://www.emergingrnleader.com/adaptive-leadership/

Spetzler, C., Winter, H., & Meyer, J. (2016). *Decision quality: Value creation from better business decisions* (1st ed.). Wiley.

Useem, M. (2010, November). Four lessons in adaptive leadership. *Harvard Business Review*.

"Creativity is intelligence having fun."
–**Albert Einstein**

5

Creativity and Innovation in a Time of Crisis

A crisis, such as the Covid-19 pandemic, is a profound existential catalyst that forces change for people worldwide. As we discussed in the previous chapter, the upheaval of previously existing systems that occurs during a crisis situation demands, at a minimum, an adaptable response that modifies pre-existing methods and practices to meet the needs of the crisis. In tandem, a crisis calls for leaders to imagine novel, creative approaches to adequately meet the demands of the crisis.

> **WE ASKED NURSE LEADERS**
>
> → When you were flying by the seat of your pants, can you identify one thing you did to deal with the crisis?
>
> → What kinds of gaps in planning became apparent as a result of responding to Covid-19?

Throughout the Covid-19 crisis, nurse leaders solved problems in creative and innovative ways. They developed new approaches and changed systems. Each day, they drove adaptation amid chaos. Drawing from their experiences, we'll hear how nurse leaders solved problems with creative and innovative solutions with IV pumps, finding space for Covid-positive patients, creating models to build Covid-compliant competencies for nurses, and delivering safe and effective care for Covid patients.

In this chapter, we will explore how nurse leaders were able to inspire and harness creativity and innovation to assist their organizations in meeting the demands of the pandemic.

CREATION AND INNOVATION IN A CRISIS

Creativity and innovation lie at the heart of crisis leadership but are each distinct concepts that should be differentiated. *Creativity* refers to the ability to create or bring something into existence. It hails from the Latin word *creare,* which means "to make, bring forth, produce, procreate, beget, cause" (Online Etymology Dictionary, n.d.). Creativity is bringing forth new ideas. At its core, creativity is subjective and very hard to measure and quantify. While the terms "innovate" and "innovation" are often used interchangeably with "create" and "creativity," the correct understanding is that innovation is the ability to take the creative idea and manifest it into reality or to make changes to something that has already been established (Govindarajan & Trimble, 2010). Whereas creativity is subjective, innovations are objective and measurable. Innovations are the products or processes that are adapted to meet the demands of a dramatic shift in reality or a crisis, necessarily employing creative ideas.

Creativity has only been recognized and valued as a core leadership skill in the past 20 years (Puccio et al., 2010). Creativity requires curiosity, unconventional and visionary thinking, open-mindedness, willingness to take risks and potentially fail, and continual experimentation (Puccio et al., 2010; van Dijk et al., 2017).

Creativity expert Robert Beghetto (2021) defines a crisis as "an experience of profound uncertainty coupled with a sense of urgency to take action to minimize or avoid potential negative outcomes" (p. 2). It is amid this "profound uncertainty" that creative thoughts materialize, requiring leaders to imagine creative solutions when the constructs they have been comfortable with no longer serve the organization or group that they are leading. Beghetto introduces a model that, although untested, provides a framework for taking creative action in times of crisis. Beghetto traces two pathways one can take when responding to a crisis that ultimately lead to a creative outcome, a deferential outcome, or a combination of the two.

First, Beghetto asserts that "creative confidence" is a necessary prerequisite to taking a creative action. If an individual possesses creative confidence, they will likely be willing to take a "creative risk," which is the next step towards creative action in Beghetto's Model. When an individual has both creative confidence and a willingness to take creative risks, they will subsequently take a creative action, which may range from highly localized (e.g., within a single group or department) to organizational to societal or even global in scale. Taking creative action does not guarantee that the action is successful or sustainable, and it is therefore important to monitor and continuously evaluate the intended and unintended consequences and subsequent impacts of the creative action.

On the flipside, if an individual does not possess creative confidence, Beghetto (2021) asserts that they will move along the deferential pathway towards a deferential outcome. An individual moving along this pathway will defer or look to others for guidance during the crisis; at its least beneficial, deferential action may result in an individual denying the crisis and/or taking no action at all. Deferential actions may also be the appropriate course of action and involve adopting subject-matter expert guidelines, such as the Centers for Disease Control recommendations in the case of the Covid crisis. Crisis leadership requires an inherent creative confidence and willingness to both take risks and evaluate those risks to determine if creative action or deferential action is the best response amid a crisis situation. Figure 5.1 illustrates Beghetto's creative action framework.

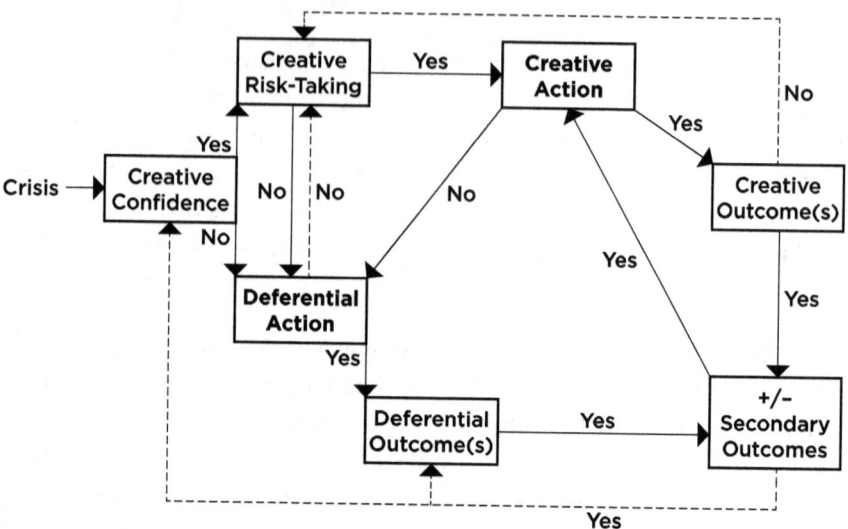

FIGURE 5.1 Beghetto's creative action framework (Beghetto, 2021).

A creative and/or innovative solution or idea does not guarantee that it will be successful, and leaders during a crisis must be willing to accept the trial-and-error nature of creative solutions and innovations. Having a solid understanding of the culture that one leads is critical in determining the proclivity for creative confidence, creative risk-taking, and creative action. This resignation for trials of innovative ideas that succeed at times and at other times need further work was acknowledged by Andrew:

> "Our culture is one of . . . I won't say perfection . . . but we certainly aren't a culture of putting something out there that hasn't been fully vetted and well prepared. We had to do some things that were just necessary but not perfect. And that was really stressful because you would work on something, you'd get it out there and then you'd have to rework on it because it wasn't perfect."
>
> Andrew, Chief Quality Officer in Nursing

CREATIVE LEADERSHIP

van Dijk, Davidson, and Mecozzi have proposed that creative leadership is both a philosophy and an action of a leader. Creative leadership "develops and realizes innovative ideas through the shared ambition of improving the world through enterprise formation. Those who employ creative leadership do so by forging an environment that promotes innovative thinking and mission-driven entrepreneurship" (van Dijk et al., 2017, p. 1). Creative leadership is a commitment to seek opportunity everywhere and embrace change. As a philosophy, it supports collaboration and supports the creativity of contributors; "through a generous, inclusive purpose deeply rooted in pragmatic idealism and empathy, it gives rise to a transcendent consciousness that goes beyond individual gratification" (van Djik et al., 2017, p. 1). As an action, creative leadership is the conceptualizing term for building effective change through dreaming big, employing innovative strategies, experimenting, and taking bold actions.

Creative leadership encourages, develops, supports, and nurtures an environment that allows new ideas to come into existence. Creative leadership encourages risk-taking, open-mindedness, going against the grain, unconventional thinking, experimentation, and failure to stay open to possible new creations, systems, and ideas. Additionally, creative leadership encourages collaboration with a holistic, universal system perspective where ideas and solutions fit into the larger picture and ideally offer benefit beyond the individual or organization and extend to societal and ecological levels (Puccio et al., 2010; van Dijk et al., 2017; Vernooij & Wolfe, 2014).

WEAVING CREATIVITY INTO LEADERSHIP THEORY

To provide a context for understanding creative leadership, it helps to review the traditional leadership theories (Table 5.1) and understand how the constructs of creative leadership can be interwoven.

Leadership theories help to frame how and why certain people become leaders. A theory is a supposition or a system of ideas intended to explain something, in this case how leaders are effective. Looking back over history, leadership was something originally believed to be inherited or inborn. More recent history asserts that leadership can be learned and the skills practiced and perfected as opposed to traits that are showcased. In many ways, specific theories allow for an understanding of the setting of the story; some businesses require more transactional relationships between leaders and subordinates, while in other industries, those that employ highly talented and motivated individuals, the setting should allow for more sharing, transformative building, and creativity. The various leadership theories help us understand how various types of businesses and industries with various levels of employee skill and participation have thrived and which have failed.

Common threads/themes include self-awareness, self-inquiry, and the relationship and shared vision between leader and follower. Clearly, some leadership theories are more amenable to inclusion of creative leadership philosophy and actions than others.

TABLE 5.1 Leadership Theories (Dass, 2008)

Leadership Theory	Description	Inclusion of Creative Leadership
Great Man Theory of Leadership (1840s)	The oldest leadership theory postulates that only men could be great leaders, utilizing the natural traits they were born with and their unique leadership qualities.	Creativity is only included as a component of the greatness exuded by the leader, who himself may be creative, but fails to inspire or acknowledge creativity within subordinates.
Trait Theory of Leadership (1930–1940s)	Great leaders have specific abilities, personal traits, and motivators which allow them to be successful.	Notably, creativity is included in the list of personal traits, but only the creativity of the leader, similar to the Great Man Theory.

Behavioral Theories of Leadership (1940–1950s)	Several smaller theories can be grouped together as behavioral theories of leadership. In these, the leader conditions their behavior for the response to any given situation: autocratic to democratic behavior to laissez-faire. Leaders subscribing to behavioral theories are focused on tasks and/or people. Situational Theory is one such sub-theory, asserting the leader adapts to the situation using one of four primary leadership styles (telling, selling, participating, delegating) per the readiness level of subordinates. The commonality is that the leader regulates their behavior based on the needs of the subordinates. Decision-making style is a component of Behavioral Leadership and includes the four distinct styles used in making decisions: collective, democratic, autocratic, and consensus. Democratic, also known as Participative, is well studied and valued as an ideal. Key to behavioral theory is that the traits of the leader can be developed and are not just innate.	Inspiring, valuing, and rewarding creativity among subordinates is only at the higher levels of behavioral theory, for those deemed more mature, self-directed, and self-actualized. Creativity, as an action, shifts from something the leader employs (in autocratic and telling/selling styles) to something the leader promotes in employees at the delegating, democratic, or laissez-faire stages.
Contingency Theory of Leadership (1960s)	Developed by Fred Fielder in 1958, Contingency Theory postulates that leaders focus on tasks (deadlines and processes) and/or relationships (people), modifying their style based on the situation and the person. Building on trait theory, this theory postulates that the employee has certain natural traits that can be capitalized on.	Creativity is employed similar to Behavioral Theory in that the leader adjusts expectations for creativity in exemplary employees, not those for whom a more task-oriented approach is necessary.

continues

TABLE 5.1 Leadership Theories (Bass, 2008) (Cont.)

Leadership Theory	Description	Inclusion of Creative Leadership
Transactional Theory of Leadership	Developed by Max Weber and Bernard M. Bass, the basis of the theory is the concept of rewards and punishments. This relationship between leader and subordinates is based on the recognition of the leader's power to perform certain tasks and reward or punish the team for their performance. The team agrees to follow the leader to accomplish a specified goal in exchange for rewards. This type of leadership fosters experimentation but also significant competition as employees vie to have the best product.	Creativity can best be employed in the experimentation stage of Transactional Leadership Theory, supporting risk-taking. What may be missing is the collaboration, nurturing, and support that are often lacking in competitive environments fostered by transactional relationships.
Transformational Theory of Leadership	This theory's foundation is the relationship between the leader and the group. Developed by expert James MacGregor Burns, trust of subordinates is developed by building quality relationships, with leaders demonstrating key components of charisma, individualized consideration, inspiration, and intellectual stimulation.	Because the leader and follower share a connection and purpose, the followers are motivated to operate on behalf of the shared idea/ideal moving beyond their own self-interest and culminating in a positive impact to society as a whole. The transformational leader raises the consciousness of both themselves and those who follow and share their vision; the transformational leader ignites intrinsic motivation within the followers, and this in turn accelerates creativity and change.

Leadership style refers to a leader's behaviors or actions when providing direction, motivation, guidance, and management of people. Most people are familiar with the autocratic leadership style in which the leader is focused primarily on results and efficiencies and retains the power to make most decisions. We tend to see these types of leaders retrospectively in industrial history within the Great Man Theory of leadership, those with the "right traits," and often military leaders. Clearly some leadership theories are more aligned with certain leadership styles.

Different historical theories recognize somewhere between five and ten distinct leadership styles. We've distilled these down to the seven most distinct. Using these industrial leadership theories, professionals develop their own style of leadership based on factors like experience and personality, as well as the unique organizational climate. As a leader develops over time, they may adopt different styles and may consciously alter their leadership style based on the needs of those they are leading and the situation to maximize their effectiveness. In addition to autocratic/authoritative, recognized leadership styles include authoritative/visionary, relationship-focused, laissez-faire, pacesetter, democratic/transformational, and transactional. Some have argued that one style or another is better, but these theories explicate that each style has a certain time and place, and a courageous leader can learn and adapt their style. Table 5.2 provides definitions and traits, and strengths and weaknesses to differentiate these historic leadership styles.

TABLE 5.2 Leadership Styles (Bass, 2008)

Leadership Style	Definition and Traits	Strengths and Weaknesses
Autocratic	Autocratic leaders are extremely experienced and strong leaders who make quick decisions with little input or consultation from their employees.	**Strengths**: Quick thinkers, great at delegating, giving directions, or making decisions in an emergency. **Weaknesses**: May not hear or value other opinions.

continues

TABLE 5.1 Leadership Styles (Bass, 2008) (Cont.)

Leadership Style	Definition and Traits	Strengths and Weaknesses
Authoritative/ Visionary	A confident leader who maps the way and sets expectations, while engaging and energizing followers along the way.	**Strengths**: Visionary leaders help others understand the direction of the company and how to achieve the objectives. They take the time to explain directives and allow staff choice and latitude on how to achieve common goals. **Weaknesses**: Similar to the weaknesses of the autocratic leader, the authoritative or visionary leader may not consider others' opinions, and could have the tendency to share goals with intent to coerce cooperation.
Relationship Focused (also called Servant, Coaching, or Affiliative)	These leaders are relationship-oriented and focus on individuals' needs. These leaders ensure employees have the skills, tools, and resources they need to achieve goals. They are highly involved in employee development and believe everyone can reach their full potential if given a little direction and support.	**Strengths**: Patient and empathetic, these leaders create goal-driven environments focused on developing their staff. **Weaknesses**: May value employee growth over task achievement.
Laissez-faire	Minimal supervision and take a "hands-off" approach. While they promote creativity and ingenuity, most change will be employee driven and thus may not keep pace with evidence-based or safety norms.	**Strengths**: Allows experienced, highly competent staff to be creative and self-managed. **Weaknesses**: Do not have an understanding of day-to-day operations nor do they promote change. May be viewed as aloof and disengaged.

Pacesetter	Highly motivated leaders who effectively set high expectations for productivity and quick change.	**Strengths**: Highly productive themselves, can quickly identify top performers and weed out those with low productivity, driving improved business results. They will pitch in and work side-by-side with staff to complete daunting tasks. **Weaknesses**: May have unrealistic expectations, causing employee distress and creating a negative work/life imbalance.
Democratic/ Transformational	Highly visionary, these leaders build engaged teams and excel at facilitating significant change. They facilitate collaborative processes, encouraging feedback, involvement, and communication from team members. They are focused on team success.	**Strengths**: Good facilitators and developers, these leaders excel in mentoring, instilling trust, building confidence, and encouraging teamwork while encouraging nurses to grow and act independently. **Weaknesses**: May be reluctant to make timely decisions independently.
Transactional	Transactional leaders are task-oriented and use a reward and punishment system to effect rapid change.	**Strengths**: Transactional leaders do well with problem-solving to meet short-term goals. Focus is on standardization and evidence-based approach to care, typically within tight deadlines and emergency situations. **Weaknesses**: The leader needs to be careful to make employees feel heard, valued, and prompted to involve creativity in their part of task resolution.

Creative leadership expands on the previously recognized styles by incorporating the necessary self-awareness and self-development of authentic leadership, the moral compass and igniting of intrinsic motivation inherent in transformational leadership, and the focus on equitable solutions and empowerment characteristics of servant leadership. Creative leadership, at its core, imagines solutions that are holistic in nature in that they benefit the organization, the organization's impact on the community and the environment, and are profitable and scalable for the organization. Creative leadership is collaborative, not competitive in nature, and it embraces the trial-and-error process knowing that creative solutions can only emerge through continual education, experimentation, risk-taking, and learning from failures (van Dijk et al., 2017).

THE THNK SCHOOL OF CREATIVE LEADERSHIP

The THNK School of Creative Leadership presents four phases of creative leadership:

1. Exploring
2. Architecting
3. Conducting
4. Directing

As previously discussed, a creative leader must remain open-minded and unconventional in their approach to problem-solving; this open-mindedness is a hallmark of the exploring phase. However, as a leader homes in on a specific approach, they must enter the more focused, tunnel-vision phase of architecting. This dichotomy of moving from an open-minded to a more narrowly focused state causes some inherent tension in creative leadership. Once a new idea or approach is outlined, the leader must again walk a fine line between directing the new idea and supporting the team to take the vision as its own and develop it from the ground up (Ball, 2014). This dance between leading from the front (conducting) and then moving to push from the back (directing) echoes the theories of transformational and servant leadership in that the leader is able to present a new idea and then motivate the team members (followers) to get on board with this idea and make it their own. The creative leader may take on some servant leadership qualities as they empower their team and give them the tools to expand on the idea, bringing in the strengths and skill sets of all the team members so that a new vision can become fully realized by the whole team. The creative leader may plant the seed, but it is the team that allows the seed to grow, flower, and fruit.

CREATIVITY DEPENDS ON A SOLID FOUNDATION

When a crisis situation like a pandemic emerges, leaders must first assess the practices and principles that are foundational to their organization and mission; these practices and principles are usually established long before the crisis occurs, and they provide a framework for imagining creative solutions. In the previous chapter on adaptability and decision-making, we touched on the need for learning from the past and having a plan for crises. But here we are delving down to the absolute basics and how that guides our inherent practice. How do we derive creative and innovative solutions to an ever-evolving set of problems?

Borrowing from architecture and building principles, the most enduring yet ornate structures all have at their base a structurally sound yet complicated foundation. While the design elements that often make a cathedral breathtaking and majestic were created by artisans with imaginative license, the cornerstones and subterranean footings were constructed and assembled by master masons or structural engineers who understood physics and structural principles. The value and safeguarding of these foundational principles were so critical that a secret brotherhood developed in the Middle Ages, riddled with mystery over this important craft. Similarly, creativity in business or healthcare can only be employed when a solid foundation has been set that fosters trust, common shared vision, standardization of procedures, and open communication among employees and leadership.

In our interviews trying to understand how creativity was fostered and employed during the Covid crisis, we observed three foundational constructs in organizations or units that were highly creative and fostered creativity:

1. Shared commitment to mission, vision, and values
2. Mutual trust and valuing expertise
3. Identifying and utilizing various leadership styles

SHARED COMMITMENT TO MISSION, VISION, AND VALUES

Foremost among those successful in employing creativity was a commitment to a shared vision or principles that transcended throughout the organization from C-suite to the front lines, from VP to Director, to Manager, to Charge Nurse. Having established priorities, guiding principles, and a shared operating commitment allows for the development of creative and innovative solutions that build on this foundation. Effective leaders and organizations nurture and value creativity in times of calm, allowing for growth even in times of stress.

If the mantra and the commitment of the organization is "safety first," then new ideas, even those generated in a crisis state, will first be judged for conforming to the undergirding obligation to safety. This commitment to the safety of the employees was verbalized by several leaders. From Kimberly, Nurse Anesthetist and Nursing Faculty:

> "The most important thing we can do is to keep our healthcare workers well. If our healthcare workers get sick, there's no one to take care of the sick patients. Keeping everyone safe translated to supplying adequate PPE and making sure that they don't get exposed. In all of the craziness and looking at all the stuff that was coming out, it's so basic: Keep your healthcare workers from getting sick. A typical example of that is they made the decision, across the board, regarding codes. This was in the early stages, if Covid status was unknown or positive and there was a cardiac arrest on the floor, they would not ventilate the patient, they would only do CPR."
>
> Kimberly, Nurse Anesthetist and Nursing Faculty

Safety of staff and the clients was also foremost in the mind of Amber, who worked in nontraditional settings with children and felt the need for connectedness with her clients. These programs were founded on creating connections and relationships that help children overcome and cope with significant health issues. Safety was clearly a priority, but assuring delivery of care that fostered their underlying mission of connectednesss was paramount:

"The first thing that I think about is the safety and well-being of our children, our families, and then of our staff. So I think it's that, again, that nursing state of mind, safety first."

Amber, Nurse Entrepreneur and Associate Professor

Amber went on to describe how having safety at the core of problem-solving allowed for her and her team to think creatively:

"And then the thing that drives me, that motivates me with everything that I do . . . [is] those connections, and that milieu, that community. How can we maintain that in this environment, with safety? I made sure that's how I looked at both programs: How can we maintain our connection with those kids? And what does that mean? Ultimately, we ended up sending massive boxes of things for the kids, their T-shirts, and all the things that they will do while they're in virtual camp; just really thinking creatively. But again, that's the team: they're acting on that vision of maintaining that connection."

Amber, Nurse Entrepreneur and Associate Professor

Another example of a deep-rooted commitment was demonstrated by a few of the medical centers regarding professional governance. It was critical to one organization that this institutional value be assured and even shored-up during a crisis. Because this commitment for professional governance and engagement was central to their practice, it was critical that the professionals, and not just the leaders, were actively engaged in the decision-making process for the institution. These leaders described intentionally not making decisions for the nursing staff on how to create more ICU beds but relying on the professional practice council to determine the best course of action.

> "We needed to create more ICU beds . . . and so I worked with our experienced staff and unit leaders to create a makeshift critical care course, using the Society of Critical Care Medicine framework. We took the PACU and part of the step-down unit and put critical care patients in there and doubled our ICU capacity by using those beds."
>
> Michelle, Innovation and Advancement Coordinator

Michelle went on to describe how the Critical Care and PACU educators worked together to capitalize on the strengths and quickly train to fill the gaps for nurses in these different areas. But the underlying principle supporting this effort was that it was run through the professional practice council to enable them to brainstorm, evaluate, modify, and then disseminate this innovative attempt throughout the system. This particular healthcare system had and maintained an institutional commitment to engage staff in not just doing the work but also in directing the change and innovating solutions through the continuation of professional practice governance.

MUTUAL TRUST AND VALUING EXPERTISE

Additionally, this same healthcare system also valued our second foundational construct for fostering creativity and innovation, extending beyond appreciating employees to assuring mutual trust and valuing expertise. Despite the premise of every thriller written, viable creative solutions don't come from someone who is a novice in the field. Creativity and innovation come from those who fully understand the situation, the nuances, and the daily operations. This in part supports professional practice governance. But it also suggests that during a crisis, experts specific for that situation need to be at the table with those directing care so that the best course can be charted.

Andrew, Chief Quality Officer in Nursing, captured this reliance on subject matter experts coupled with the commitment for professional governance as a cornerstone for innovation. In particular, note the language involved and the assumption of a transformative leadership style, trusting the experts and team with innovative decisions:

> "The pace of work changed and my role changed from being in the weeds of it to being a facilitator for the subject matter experts, giving them the power and the authority to come up with innovative solutions, rather than me. I realized the strength of my people and that they were fully competent. Not that I didn't know this before, but I realized I didn't have to always be dealing with the details, and it's really changed how I interact with them. There's more trust. I'm more confident in the team's ability to solve problems. It's helped me grow as a leader as well, giving them more autonomy and authority and reliance on what their expertise is. That's what they do. And that's what they do every day."
>
> Andrew, Chief Quality Officer in Nursing

A firm foundation of trust between leadership and staff is necessary to navigate daily operations and essential in times of crisis. Daily operations and quality improvement are fraught with change, and how management leads employees through these types of activities—valuing input, reinforcing ownership, fostering creativity—is absolutely essential for constructing a foundation of trust. Employees need to believe that changes and innovations they develop and work to implement are actually realized, including navigating any pushback to those changes. Further, there needs to be a level of trust that allows for the reset of actions for both employees and leadership. At every level during the early days of the pandemic, organizations struggled with not knowing the right approach and having to learn via trial and error and from the observations of others. While there was grumbling about the reversal of policies related to PPE, cleaning, isolation, and delivery of care, no large-scale mutinies occurred because leadership had foundational trust with employees that processes were being trialed in full transparency as they navigated unchartered waters together. From Sidney, Federally Qualified Health Center Nursing Director:

> "There [are] a lot of policies that changed as we learned more about the disease, and I think a big part of change management is communicating those policy changes and maintaining a sense of trust. And I think a lot of people lost trust because they didn't understand why the policies were changing as we learned more about Covid being airborne and things like that . . . I think that's a key leadership point of knowing how frequently you need to repeat the messages you're sharing and how much you need to justify and explain why if everyone's in crisis mode. If a leader is in crisis mode and they're just saying do this and not telling why, you're not going to have trust for long. So I think that's definitely something that takes a lot of time and effort to help maintain that trust, as you change your messaging and [procedures]."
>
> Sidney, Federally Qualified Health Center Nursing Director

IDENTIFYING AND UTILIZING A VARIETY OF LEADERSHIP STYLES

The third construct, which must be foundational, harkens back to the first discussion in this chapter related to identifying and valuing the various leadership styles. In our experience, creativity flourishes in particular leadership styles. Reading back over the various leadership theories and styles, it may be tempting to identify one as being the best or the ideal that should always be employed by great leaders. Quite certainly, transformational leaders have been identified during times of prosperity and growth as leading in a way that builds trust with, engages, and values employees. It also facilitates creativity and ingenuity; however, one of the biggest criticisms is the inability to make rapid, critical decisions in an emergency. Often, leaders will adopt more of an authoritarian or autocratic leadership style during a crisis, or one who has this innate style will step forward and assume command. A successful organization will employ and develop a treasure trove of leaders with various styles, maturity levels, and abilities, allowing the organization to pivot and restructure some aspects of leadership to implement an Incident Command System, appropriately delegate, employ creativity to handle various situations, and make key decisions.

Foundational is that the organization has an emergency response plan developed, articulating and updating the various roles with the appropriate leader based on their leadership styles and traits. This certainly could be done superficially with plugging in a VP in this role. We suggest that a more thoughtful approach would be to use leadership trait inventories and validated measures to help identify the various competences and strengths of the leadership team and assign these roles accordingly. This takes foundational work prior to any crisis and then should be followed up with exercises and mock scenarios to allow for safe role rehearsal. This also requires that the senior leadership team fully engage with their middle management, understanding and valuing each unique contribution. The differences in leadership style should be celebrated and further developed.

Finally, inherent within this understanding of the various leaders and styles is the acceptance and buy-in from the individual leaders that their role may well change. They must have the maturity, flexibility, and mental mindset to view challenges as "windows of opportunity," relinquishing control and trusting team members to each contribute. Our interviews revealed many of these concepts. Carson, the Vice President of Nursing Practice and Education, discussed changing the focus of his role from being task-oriented prior to Covid and having to stop work on regular projects and focus more on staff:

"Covid has certainly changed my role, and it has changed the roles of lots of leaders because we had our regular workflows, we had the regular projects that we were supporting and building, and then with Covid, all of a sudden we had to think very differently about PPE and about staffing—about safety of our teams."

Carson, Vice President of Nursing Practice and Education

Symone, Education Coordinator for the NICU, described becoming more relationship-focused and being servant-focused with being present and available for her nursing staff:

"I changed my leadership to be more present with my staff . . . I found that I did a lot of my work inside the unit, just so I could be there with them as they're going through trying to manage and take care of the patients that we put on isolation. I could be immediately available to them if they had any questions, or I could just jump up and watch them don their PPE, or when they come out [of] the room, making sure they're doffing it correctly. So yes, it was a definite change from my everyday routine. I didn't wear normal dress clothes anymore; I wore scrubs every day. I kind of switched my office to the unit to allow me to multitask [so] I could be in there and then also [work] on my other things at the same time."

Symone, Education Coordinator for NICU

Observations of Andrew (Chief Quality Officer in Nursing) regarding the authority of incident command, delegation, and leadership roles:

"We had groups that were given the authority and the permission to make recommendations and decisions based on their subject matter expertise, with the command center deferring to their expertise and just [weighing] in on whether or not there were unintended consequences of those decisions. But if there weren't unintended consequences then they came in and said, 'OK, you're the experts, go ahead and go do that.' And that was the command center's purview to make sure they had the resources, money, and the assessment of [the interventions and evaluation]. This process and identifying key people really elevated our governance and decision-making and our ability to pull people together that have the subject matter expertise to tackle whatever challenge presented."

Andrew, Chief Quality Officer in Nursing

Finally, this quote from Carson, Vice President of Nursing Practice and Education, about embracing change as an opportunity:

"All my years in management, you always want to look at if there is a window of opportunity—people see it as a problem—it's really a window of opportunity. So, what can you do to either fix it, change it, enhance it?—Not sit there and just watch it and just talk about it and just watch it spin out of control because if you do that and think, oh, somebody else can do it, then you're part of the problem, not part of the solution."

Carson, Vice President of Nursing Practice and Education

FOSTERING CREATIVITY AND INNOVATION IN A CRISIS

As healthcare organizations pivoted to crisis mode in March of 2020, in addition to the employment of foundational constructs outlined in Table 5.3, the healthcare leaders described several qualities that promoted innovative solutions to operational and patient care dilemmas. Leaders described having an open perspective and readiness to pivot and innovate on a moment's notice.

TABLE 5.3 Foundational Constructs Necessary to Allow for Creativity and Innovation During a Crisis

Construct	Examples
Shared commitment to mission, vision, and values	Commitment to safety first
	Commitment to professional governance structure
Mutual trust and valuing expertise	A firm foundation of trust between leadership and staff prior to the crisis
	Allowance for reset in actions
	Reliance on subject matter experts
	Experts in fields like epidemiologists
	Frontline employees who know care processes
Identifying and utilizing various leadership styles	Understanding own and others' leadership styles
	Thoughtful assignment to specific roles based on leadership traits
	Mindset of viewing change as an opportunity

The necessity for quick decision-making and action was described eloquently by Andrew, Chief Quality Officer in Nursing, embracing the challenges of problems, some within but others not usually in his purview:

"So we started working immediately on . . . the things within the electronic medical record that we need to change to prepare for Covid, whether it is documentation of symptoms, documentation of travel, building on some of the tools that we already had, putting in order sets for the isolation statuses for Covid, building things that would make it more visible within the electronic medical record when someone was being evaluated for Covid or was positive for Covid. And then probably the very first thing that I worked on was trying to figure out how to get Covid results back to patients. The lab ramped up Covid testing so quickly. We didn't have a process for testing so many people."

Andrew, Chief Quality Officer in Nursing

This was accompanied by the ability to make swift but innovative decisions, often acting without a solid evidence base and having to improvise. From Carson, Vice President of Nursing Practice and Education for a large healthcare system, we learned:

"Being able to actually make a decision is an important part of governance, and when you seek input and you're working on teams and there's collaboration and there is discussion at some point, I used to jokingly say, 'We've gotta pull the trigger!' We talked about this; we talked it to death. We have come at it from every particular angle, and at some point, even if you feel like you don't have all of the pieces or all of the answers, you have to make the best decision based on what you know at the time and you have to just go for it."

Carson, Vice President of Nursing Practice and Education

Kimberly, Nurse Anesthetist and Nursing Faculty, described the early decision that required rapid response of how to handle not having sufficient supply of N95 masks in the OR suites and innovating to protect other staff from the possibility of aerosolization of the Covid virus during intubation:

> "Initially the only people wearing N95s were the anesthesia providers. The other people in the room did not have N95s due to scarcity. So we had to make sure that they went out of the room when we intubated; they would have to stay out of the room for one air cycle change."
>
> Kimberly, Nurse Anesthetist and Nursing Faculty

Returning to our opening definitions, innovation was more often employed over creativity. Innovation allowed for processes that had been used with Ebola to be refined and translated, applying to the Covid virus:

> "Epidemiology and infection prevention took a tremendous leap in defining processes. For screening people at the building, they would take those processes and develop their own quick training for people to be door screeners, for PPE observations. Our serious communicable disease unit group had a lot of history with Ebola, in the management of personal protective equipment, and how to do training around the donning and doffing. So, they used that knowledge of the Ebola crisis to translate that into those Covid units and they adapted that training to that. And those people would go through that training and [be] signed off for competency before they would go there. So . . . it was really . . . a 'just in time' type of training."
>
> Andrew, Chief Quality Officer in Nursing

Similarly, resources (material, human, and systemic) were repurposed to adapt to the changing circumstances. This included quickly identifying and upscaling under-utilized resources, such as telehealth and working and hosting meetings remotely. Andrew shared how they assessed and developed "a reliable mechanism to have a provider-patient encounter over telehealth, [using] tablets or PCs with cameras." Some challenges included:

"Making sure that we had a way to schedule a visit where the patients knew it was a telehealth visit as they were showing up in person. Now around 30 to 35% of all the ambulatory encounters are telehealth visits. We also ensured through the electronic medical record to let people know if someone was Covid positive, or what the status of their result was. So we did a lot of work on those reporting mechanisms, building electronic patient lists and the medical record that identifies patients that need follow-up, adding the isolation status for Covid, and the result of the Covid test to make it highly visible."

Andrew, Chief Quality Officer in Nursing

Finally, frequent and transparent communication of creative and innovative changes was paramount. As described by Symone (Education Coordinator for NICU), communication must occur even when it is difficult and ever-changing:

"Because stuff was changing all the time, it is my goal to make sure the staff has everything they need, education-wise and how to do their job . . . I just tried my best to stay on top of information that was coming through and all the changes and making sure I communicated that out to everyone. I hate when I put something out there and then it changes the next day. But then it just got to the point, you know what, nobody knows what's going on, we just have to, this is what's happening right now, we all have to be aware of that, we're trying to get it right. But it may not be right, and it may change tomorrow. So, you take that approach to it."

Symone, Education Coordinator for NICU

In many ways, the Covid crisis brought forth more efficient and effective systems and ways of operating. Some of the learning identified in employing creativity the first year of the pandemic were hard-won and ongoing.

Leaders described the need for continual re-evaluation, along with measurement of outcomes in a systematic fashion to assure the innovation was reliable. In some situations, unforeseen outcomes or symptoms caused a rethink of an action, as relayed by Kathy, Chief Nursing Officer:

"We got really creative on some things. In the original surge, the first part of it, we converted the PACU to a Covid patient care area. Then as the numbers came down in April [2020], we went back to normal operations. With this surge in July [2020], we learned some lessons that had us rethink the PACU. With that variant, diarrhea was a much larger problem, and the PACU did not have bathrooms. So the second time around, we knew we needed more bathrooms. We cannot be relying on bedside commodes."

Kathy, Chief Nursing Officer

Several leaders who worked in large healthcare systems stressed that standardization of novel ideas in all areas was imperative. Because staff were being called to float to multiple different areas, it was critical that new procedures implemented in one area were also adopted in others:

"Changes had to be on a system level, particularly for our nurses who float between one department to another. Our unit remains the only true Covid-ICU in the system, as most have either dissolved or they are now hybrids. But a few weeks ago, we had to open some pop-up units. We had three, four, five floors that were Covid-ICUs. So the consistency of care has to remain. We cannot create a process that is used only on one unit. The processes we implemented came from [the collaboration of] Infection Disease and Prevention, Nursing, and IT. It has to come from one specific group that is managing all information, all communication, all practice for Covid patients."

Vivian, Critical Care Unit Director

Further, while creativity and innovation were embraced, as healthcare practitioners and scientists, there remained institutional commitments to engaging in the scientific method to evaluate and continuously refine new practices. This was imperative as innovations were often imperfect and required revision and refinement. Sharma, Director of Nursing Leadership, reflected:

"I think that is really the strength of the work that's been done in a number of teams. What Covid has taught us in caring for patients, as well as caring for ourselves, are frameworks that will help strengthen our organization—now but also into the future. We continue to evaluate the things that we put in place and tweak where we need to; adapt as needed, but also shore up so we can address if the science changes and make revisions."

Sharma, Director of Nursing Leadership

Finally, creative expansion as a result of crisis revealed the gaps in the systems that needed repair, reinforcement, restructuring to create stronger systems of communication, preparation, technology, and infrastructure:

"I think the hardest change that we attempted and were not successful with was this . . . Once surgeries opened back up, patients had to be tested for Covid prior to coming in. We undertook a process where we attempted to collaborate with those external testing centers so if surgery was scheduled at one place but the patient lived closer to the sister facility, they could get tested at the more convenient location. We weren't successful at doing it. For a couple of reasons, our technology infrastructure did not make the process efficient or effective, yet if we engineered a new process, it would have been so cumbersome to the clinical staff it probably would have caused more problems than it would have solved. The difficulty was communicating to staff and to leadership why something that everyone believes we should be able to do, that we all believe is the right thing to do, is not possible. The resource limitations, the technology limitations, just didn't allow it to be successful. I think that was one of the most difficult things for me because I was a co-leader on that project. Nobody likes to fail. A part of leadership, I think, is being able to fully describe why something can't work at a given time, even after you've spent a tremendous amount of time trying to make it work. We did that."

Andrew, Chief Quality Officer in Nursing

NURSING INNOVATION IN THE COVID ERA

Although before Covid-19 there were glimmers of innovation, the pandemic has unleashed the tremendous capacity of the nursing workforce to change the ways of the past (Brunson, 2021). As we have commented previously, the mobilization of nurses and other resources in record time to meet surge Covid capacities presented additional problems requiring creative solutions. Universally, innovation was demonstrated through 3D printing of PPE, expanded telehealth, staff headbands to prevent skin breakdown, and simulation training for nurses and nursing students.

Unfortunately, much that was happening centered on all of the things we "couldn't do," which was antithetical to what nurses utilize as standards of care. For example, family visitation was strictly limited when nurses were cognizant of the American Association of Critical-Care Nurses (AACN) stance on family visitation. The AACN (2016) has highlighted the evidence showing unrestricted access and participation by families can improve safety of care and communication and enhance patient and staff satisfaction. To circumvent the lack of human visitation, nurses were pulling out their personal cell phones for video calls and eventually using unit-based tablets. Nationwide, grateful patients, families, and donors were providing iPads for visitation.

Staffing changes not only involved redeployment but actual physical strategies to limit exposure. At one hospital (Brunson, 2021), medical-surgical nurses conducted bedside patient care in the ICU, while the ICU RN and the associated ICU equipment were placed outside of the patient room. Therefore, the ICU nurse could provide support to the bedside nurse while still monitoring the idiosyncrasies of the equipment. Other innovations include the use of healthcare robots, QR codes for in-service training, and specified task lists for teams.

We have highlighted throughout the book the ingenuity we heard about, witnessed, and admired, and we feel quite sure there are countless more incidents of nurse leaders committed to finding a way to simply get things done. With the ever-changing nature of the pandemic, every level of the healthcare team was pressed to continually innovate. Many of the strategies had been used in the military or on a short-term basis but were now demonstrated to be effective on a national level and can be further built on in the future.

KEY TAKEAWAYS

Creativity and innovation are essential elements in problem-solving and adapting to crises, especially one as protracted as the Covid pandemic. By definition, a crisis is an unusual and dangerous event that can overwhelm resources; thus, while some planning and preparation can be useful in mitigating the impact, often unexpected challenges are faced. Past typical responses are often inadequate for handling the present situation, and evidenced-based treatments are unknown or even unimagined. But creativity does not just simply sprout amid the chaos.

Importantly in this chapter, we discussed how there is a time and place for virtually all leadership styles, but the critical actions are to know your personal leadership style, be able to capitalize on your leadership strengths in a crisis management structure or incident command, and be willing to adapt your style to meet changing organizational needs. Successful strategies for fostering creativity and innovation along with several lessons learned were presented, which may assist others in tapping into their own leadership innovation during times of crises.

REFLECTIVE EXERCISES

5.1 → CREATIVITY AND INNOVATION SELF-ASSESSMENT

What was the most creative or innovative change you have led?

Was this change creative or innovative?

List the challenges you faced in bringing forth this change.

Is the process still being used today? Has it been evaluated, altered, or adapted to other environments?

5.2 → LEADERSHIP STYLES SELF-ASSESSMENT

Reflecting on the various leadership styles, identify which leadership style you are most productive working under and then the styles you are more likely to employ when you are leading a group based on the situation. Do you vary in your styles preferred or employed?

Situation	Preferred Style to Be Led	Employed Leadership Style
The need to adopt a new wound dressing that has been shown to decrease costs.		
The need to change practice of a critical intervention that has been shown to decrease mortality (e.g., proning in respiratory failure).		
Instituting regular monthly mock codes as a means to improve CPR outcomes with > 80% staff involvement.		

5.3 → CREATIVE LEADERSHIP INSTITUTIONAL SUPPORT ASSESSMENT

How does your current role allow you to exercise your creative leadership abilities?

_____
_____
_____
_____

How has your present employer built a foundation from which creativity can grow in both routine times and times of crisis?

_____
_____
_____
_____

5.4 → SUPPORTING OTHERS TO CREATE AND INNOVATE

Creativity also requires discipline and direction. Describe what and how you would both encourage and focus an innovative idea from a subordinate.

I would encourage innovation by:

_____
_____
_____
_____

I would encourage focus by:

_____

_____

_____

_____

What would be key factors for the implementation of this creative process in your unit?

_____

_____

_____

_____

REFERENCES

American Association of Critical-Care Nurses. (2016, February 1). Family visitation in the adult ICU. *Critical Care Nurse, 36*(1), e15–e18. https://doi.org/10.4037/ccn2016677

Ball, R. (2014). *The paradoxes of creative leadership*. https://www.thnk.org/insights/the-paradoxes-of-creative-leadership/

Bass, B. (2008). *The Bass handbook of leadership* (4th edition). Free Press.

Beghetto, R. A. (2021, January 7). How times of crisis serve as a catalyst for creative action: An agentic perspective. *Frontiers in Psychology*. https://doi.org/10.3389/fpsyg.2020.600685

Brunson, M. E. (2021). Disruptive innovation for the unstoppable nurse leader. *Nursing Management, 52*(5), 22–29. https://doi.org/10.1097/01.NUMA.0000743416.28424.37

Govindarajan, V., & Trimble, C. (2010). *The other side of innovation: Solving the execution challenge*. Harvard Business Press.

Online Etymology Dictionary. (n.d.). *Create*. https://www.etymonline.com/search?q=creare

Puccio, G. J., Mance, M., & Murdock, M. C. (2010). *Creative leadership: Skills that drive change*. Sage Publications.

van Dijk, M., Davidson, G., & Mecozzi, V. (2017). *Creative leadership.* School of Creative Leadership. https://www.thnk.org/content/uploads/2018/01/Creative-Leadership.pdf

Vernooij, M., & Wolfe, R. (2014). *The need for creative leadership.* https://www.thnk.org/insights/the-need-for-creative-leadership/

> *"I am a firm believer in the people. If given the truth, they can be depended upon to meet any national crisis. The great point is to bring them the real facts."*
> —Abraham Lincoln, 16th President of the United States

6
Multifaceted Communication

Communication is undeniably essential in all facets of our personal, familial, professional, and spiritual spheres. It is the spoken word, gestures and body positioning, laughter and tears, print and visual media, the song we can't get out of our head, the fiery passages of famous speeches that should never be forgotten. The communication of thoughts, of beliefs, of inspiration, of emotions.

The field of communications is expansive, with numerous areas of study. Countless books, theses, presentations, and educational classes have been developed on communication. How to communicate more effectively, how to be understood, how to motivate your audience, how to sell your message or product, and how to have those uncomfortable, yet crucial, conversations.

WE ASKED NURSE LEADERS

→ What strategies did you use to inform staff of changes that were occurring to prevent confusion or resistance to change?

→ What was unique about the communication of information during Covid that is different from normal circumstances?

Healthcare communication has more specific purposes related to promoting community health, outlining specific services, imparting health education, and improving health understanding and literacy. Health communication is especially seminal to multicultural societies because both culture and language create bridges and barriers to understanding health and communicating around personal and community issues of health directed to specific populations. Because of the risks to life and health, effective strategies of communication between health systems and the communities they serve and between providers and patients is critical to well-being. Incorrect information sharing or misunderstandings about health approaches and treatments can have a devastating negative effect that is not easily corrected. As seen at every stage of the Covid pandemic, communication approaches and the veracity of information shared can be easily sabotaged by inadequate or incomplete information and understanding. Effective communication in healthcare requires a firm foundation in evidence, facts, clarity, and utility (Pagano & Pagano, 2017).

The Oxford English Dictionary defines communication as "the imparting or exchanging of information by speaking, writing, or using some other medium" (OED, 2021). But communication is not just the unidirectional conveyance of information. It also involves the necessary reception and then dialogue whereby the message is validated (Parvanta & Bass, 2020). Effective communication requires the ability to listen and be present. Finally, rarely is the ultimate objective of communication the simple transmission of ideas; rather it serves to develop consensus, formulate a plan, and create. Communication is a bidirectional exchange whereby a product is conceived, developed, and born.

COMMUNICATION DURING CRISIS

While communication is the backbone of society and business during everyday life, communication during a crisis takes on new critical status. Recognized as an integral branch of public relations, crisis communication is a specialty unto itself with specific leadership, training, and responsibilities.

An early example of effective crisis communication by private business with the public is observed in Johnson & Johnson's (J&J) handling of product tampering with their Tylenol capsules, causing seven deaths in 1982. J&J immediately ran advertisements to alert consumers not to take their product, stopped production, and ordered a national withdrawal. After six weeks, they released the first triple-lock tamper-resistant container. By their immediate and transparent response to the crisis, and promoting their valuing of their customers, J&J regained its market share.

Conversely, dishonest communication and shifting the blame is remembered far longer than the actual crisis. In 2010, a BP oil rig off the Gulf Coast exploded, creating the largest oil spill in US history. An estimated 130 million gallons of oil leaked into the Gulf of Mexico, and 11 lives were lost in the initial explosion. Sadly, what is remembered is that BP was dishonest with the facts they initially released, stating that the oil rig was leaking up to 1,000 barrels of oil a day, when the real number was later found to be closer to 5,000. BP then attempted to shift the blame to the owners of the rig, Transocean Ltd., and diminish their role in the crisis.

In our national leadership, we have seen how critical communication has been employed to succinctly provide the facts, unite the country, and chart a course. A historic example of this is the speech President Roosevelt gave the day after Pearl Harbor was attacked (see the following sidebar; Roosevelt, 1941). Take the time to read this famous speech, noting the succinctness and the presentation of facts but also the underlying emotion. Take a moment to visualize how your grandparents or other distant relatives must have received this speech, from a radio in their living rooms, as this decision to enter into war was conveyed.

The President Requests War Declaration 125, "December 7, 1941, a Date Which Will Live in Infamy" Address to the Congress Asking That a State of War Be Declared Between the United States and Japan, December 8, 1941

Mr. Vice President, and Mr. Speaker, and Members of the Senate and House of Representatives:

YESTERDAY, December 7, 1941, a date which will live in infamy, the United States of America was suddenly and deliberately attacked by naval and air forces of the Empire of Japan.

The United States was at peace with that Nation and, at the solicitation of Japan, was still in conversation with its Government and its Emperor looking toward the maintenance of peace in the Pacific. Indeed, one hour after Japanese air squadrons had commenced bombing in the American Island of Oahu, the Japanese Ambassador to the United States and his colleague delivered to our Secretary of State a formal reply to a recent American message. And while this reply stated that it seemed useless to continue the existing diplomatic negotiations, it contained no threat or hint of war or of armed attack.

It will be recorded that the distance of Hawaii from Japan makes it obvious that the attack was deliberately planned many days or even weeks ago. During the intervening time the Japanese Government has deliberately sought to deceive the United States by false statements and expressions of hope for continued peace.

The attack yesterday on the Hawaiian Islands has caused severe damage to American naval and military forces. I regret to tell you that very many American lives have been lost. In addition, American ships have been reported torpedoed on the high seas between San Francisco and Honolulu.

Yesterday the Japanese Government also launched an attack against Malaya. Last night Japanese forces attacked Hong Kong. Last night Japanese forces attacked Guam. Last night Japanese forces attacked the Philippine Islands. Last night the Japanese attacked Wake Island. And this morning the Japanese attacked Midway Island.

Japan has, therefore, undertaken a surprise offensive extending throughout the Pacific area. The facts of yesterday and today speak for themselves. The people of the United States have already formed their opinions and well understand the implications to the very life and safety of our Nation.

As Commander in Chief of the Army and Navy I have directed that all measures be taken for our defense.

> But always will our whole Nation remember the character of the onslaught against us.
>
> No matter how long it may take us to overcome this premeditated invasion, the American people in their righteous might will win through to absolute victory.
>
> I believe that I interpret the will of the Congress and of the people when I assert that we will not only defend ourselves to the uttermost but will make it very certain that this form of treachery shall never again endanger us.
>
> Hostilities exist. There is no blinking at the fact that our people, our territory, and our interests are in grave danger.
>
> With confidence in our armed forces with the unbounding determination of our people we will gain the inevitable triumph so help us God.
>
> I ask that the Congress declare that since the unprovoked and dastardly attack by Japan on Sunday, December 7, 1941, a state of war has existed between the United States and the Japanese Empire.

Much has been developed regarding crisis communication to the public. A variety of training resources have been assimilated by the Department of Homeland Security at https://www.dhs.gov/science-and-technology/frg-training, including a link to the Centers for Disease Control and Prevention (CDC) comprehensive Crisis and Emergency Risk Communication (CERC) manual, which "provides an evidence-based framework and best practices for anyone who communicates on behalf of an organization responding to a public health emergency" (CDC, 2018, p. 2). An extensive library of training tools and components of this manual is online at https://emergency.cdc.gov/cerc/manual/index.asp and is highly valuable for all leaders to study.

THE SIX GUIDING PRINCIPLES OF CRISIS COMMUNICATION

While most organizations will designate a specific spokesperson for public communication on behalf of the company, all leaders should understand the basics provided here and employ the CERC's six main principles of crisis and emergency communication (CDC, 2018):

- Be first
- Be right
- Be credible
- Express empathy
- Promote action
- Show respect

Before continuing, page back to President Roosevelt's speech. Identify these crucial elements of communication.

Beyond communication with the public, our nursing leaders utilized these same communication tactics when communicating with their stakeholders, most often their direct subordinates or populations served.

BE FIRST

> *"Make sure to communicate your idea quickly and keep it straight to the point."*
> –Paul Bailey, author

Timeliness is the first tenet. Crises are time-sensitive, and communicating information quickly is crucial. With the Covid-19 pandemic and healthcare response, most leaders reported participating in daily (or twice/thrice daily!) command center meetings and then disseminating critical information to their employees through daily huddles. The objective was to assure timely communication of critical information to address needs, empower employees, and squash rumors.

"When we stood up, I was attending the command center huddle twice a day, seven days a week, so that I made sure I had the right information. Even though we're getting tons of emails, I relied on those huddles to make sure that I was accurately understanding what was being passed. Then I would have huddles with my team to try to pass on that information and to answer their questions, while at the same time they're giving me questions that I can pass back up to the huddle that I'm attending."

Andrew, Chief Quality Officer in Nursing

Repeatedly, we heard from leaders about *tiered huddles* as one of the most effective forms of communication. At the top of an organization was the executive level team, often termed the Command Center or C-Suite Huddle. In most of our interviewed leaders' organizations, this high-level team met two to three times a day during the initial days of the pandemic and then with the surges that occurred over the past 20 months. From there, the leaders huddled with their direct reports and from there, those leaders to units. The frequency and timelines of these huddles allowed for not just the unidirectional communication of directives but also bidirectional communication of ideas and concerns, filtered up and down.

BE RIGHT

"Fast is fine, but accuracy is everything. In a gunfight . . . you need to take your time in a hurry."
–Wyatt Earp, lawman in the Old West

Critical to this communication is accuracy, as expressed in the second command: to be right. As outlined by the CDC, accuracy establishes credibility. Information needs include not just what is known but also what is not known and what is being done to fill in the gaps. With this pandemic, the rapidity of changes in care was often unsettling to healthcare providers. Men and women who had cut their teeth on evidence-based practice and Cochrane Systematic Reviews were now having to make decisions and trust small samples and observational conclusions. Our care was directed from fighting similar viruses and hypothesized best treatments. Protocols were changed overnight. It simply was doing the best we could; however, it was often trial and re-adjust—not trial and error but small readjusting approaches and treatments for what worked for one patient and how to apply to 10,000 more.

Nancy, a Critical Care Clinical Nurse Specialist, summarized this rapid-fire change utilizing limited data:

"There was one study that came out of Europe with maybe 30,000 patients, which is a hefty number of people, it's a good size. They found that patients who got on steroids were more likely to survive, and it was published somewhere like the *European Journal of Clinical Microbiology & Infectious Diseases* or *International Journal of Infectious Diseases*, a big journal. All of a sudden, out of nowhere the United States sunk their teeth into one big fat observational study! Which they tell you in evidence-based practice class, never sink your teeth into one study, and certainly not a randomized control trial, right? Well, we did! And it's actually been working out really, really well! So, everybody, pretty much everybody, goes on dexamethasone now, Decadron. So that was another source of our data as well, what is coming out of the whole world as we struggle with this."

Nancy, Critical Care Clinical Nurse Specialist

Aside from the fact that nurses and physicians were now making decisions based on nontraditional research methods and were instead relying on observational data, actions were further designated based on their significant and heart-wrenching experiences with patients, many of whom died. This was difficult for healthcare providers but ground shaking for the public, who could not grasp that we were not unified in a consensus treatment for something that was literally life-threatening. Leaders often discussed how it was important to openly discuss the latest research, put forth alternative thoughts based on what they were experiencing, and then, as a collective, make a decision related to implementation.

"Things change every day, so we [had] a 15-minute huddle on what the latest and greatest information was. And this was led primarily by the attending who was working in the unit that day—they would cover for a week at a time. We also had Friday huddles at 1:30 with the attending and anybody else who wanted to join to talk about what the science is, what we know today, how we have to change our protocols."

Nancy, Critical Care Clinical Nurse Specialist

Kimberly, Nurse Anesthetist and Nursing Faculty for a large hospital system, described:

"To get this huge group of people to essentially change what they're doing was very difficult. And just like we saw with the CDC over the course of the initial outbreak, one day we would say, 'OK, we're going to do it this way.' And then something would come out two days later and we'd say, 'No, no, no, no, no! Don't do it like that!' And we'd have to then communicate this reversal . . . it was extremely frustrating."

Kimberly, Nurse Anesthetist and Nursing Faculty

Vital to being accurate is having the experts sharing their knowledge and informing the care decisions that are made. Just as the White House conducted briefings with the eminent leaders in public health and epidemiology, it was important for healthcare workers on the front lines to have access to similar experts:

> "We set up dedicated time for Q&A, which they called Town Hall sessions, where people could come and the leaders from all organizations would be available. The [leaders were the] CEO, CNO, the epidemiologists, and infection prevention [experts] for the various hospitals. During these sessions, you could see the anxiety on the [faces of] employees . . . it didn't matter where you worked. In these Town Hall sessions, you could ask any number of questions, hear the most up-to-date information. Similarly, we relied heavily on our infectious disease champions, our ID docs, and we had direct access to the CDC."
>
> Sharma, Director of Nursing Leadership

BE CREDIBLE

"When the trust account is high, communication is easy, instant, and effective."
–Stephen R. Covey, author and professional speaker

While being accurate is paramount, being credible may be even more important. Honesty and truthfulness cannot be compromised during crises, including being transparent when the correct direction or course of action is not known. As a collective, clinicians don't often like to admit that they don't have the answer, but with Covid, accepting the uncertainty and being transparent about what was known and unknown were the best steps forward.

"Because in the beginning, nobody knew! The CDC really didn't know . . . we didn't know if mothers with Covid should be separated from their newborn babies. My team works with breastfeeding, and we didn't have any information on whether they should breastfeed or not. We knew that with influenza, [the virus] is not in the breast milk, and early studies [with Covid-19] didn't show it in the breast milk, so we thought that maybe they should just wash their hands and wear a mask. We're really used to being able to go to books, professional journals, and websites, but at the beginning of this, there was nobody to tell us because no one knew! So, we put together a sheet that basically said this is what we know, this is what we think we know, this is what we have no idea about yet."

Tanja, Unit Director Labor and Delivery

"So, whenever I heard anything, I wanted to be able to pass that on to the people in the teams that I have been working with because it was really important to be as transparent as possible. But being clear, as of right now, at this time, this is the message. It is not written in stone and quite possibly may change at any given moment. But for right now, this is the information we have. I think communicating that way, instead of waiting until we had more clarity around the communication, helped us take action and build reliability."

Vivian, Critical Care Unit Director

Part of being a credible leader is assuring that you are contributing to the credibility of the organization or institution you serve. Clearly the rumors that can circulate during any crisis can quickly overcome the best of intentions or the clearest of communication. We were impressed with this tactic used by one of the nursing leaders we interviewed to tackle rumors directly:

"So, we had tons of emails flying around: lots of rumors, questions, phone calls. One of the questions I ask at every one of my huddles is, if there is any new information or any rumors that anybody needs to bring up today that you heard [which were] different from yesterday? And that way, we were able to just discuss it. Given the opportunity for people to just speak up and say, 'I'm confused; I don't know what to do, help me out,' we were able to directly address or go find out the information and get back with them."

Andrew, Chief Quality Officer in Nursing

Finally, part of being credible is recognizing that mistakes were made and that communication may have failed. Despite our best intentions, when we think we have all bases covered and all questions answered so that we can implement a strategy system-wide, sometimes the failure to launch was not with the intervention so much as the lack of clear and effective communication surrounding it. Failing to oversee every step of this communication in rolling out a new strategy is a hard lesson to learn and accept responsibility for.

"What are other weaknesses? Learning the communication structures, assuming that we've made this decision, we're going to communicate it with these groups, and assuming that was enough. And then we'd roll something out, thinking it's rolled out and then a week later it's still not happening because I didn't help guide the communication, the way it needed to go."

Carson, Vice President of Nursing Practice and Education

EXPRESS EMPATHY

"It's important to make sure that we're talking with each other in a way that heals, not in a way that wounds."
—Barack Obama, US President

As touched on earlier, communication is bi-directional and involves listening—not just to what is said but to the emotions felt and the challenges being faced by the team. The pandemic created fear, extremes in working conditions, short-staffing, anguish, illness, and even death. For nurses and every healthcare worker, every communication, every decision, and every shortage was surrounded by some emotion, and the effective leader needed to be able to acknowledge and effectively guide and even manage this emotion when possible. Leaders handled this differently depending on their situation and audience. For some it was being as prepared and informed as possible:

> "When you go in every day, you have to make sure that you don't bring that same level of anxiety that they're already experiencing. They don't need that. They need leadership that is well educated and informed. I made sure I was on top of everything that was sent through, communication-wise. I was very cognizant to make sure I read what was sent through emails every day before I stepped into that unit so I could answer every single question. I felt like I needed to be prepared for my staff when they came to me with those questions. So, I will say I did step up my game so far as making sure I knew what was going on at all times."
>
> Symone, Education Coordinator for NICU

Similarly, our leaders made certain they had the best information possible:

"It makes me emotional thinking about it because it was so overwhelming, and we felt such a responsibility to make sure that we had the best information that we had to give to our people who were out there working."

Kimberly, Nurse Anesthetist and Nursing Faculty

Several times, we heard how leaders acknowledged being available, present, and vulnerable to their staff as a necessary component of compassionate and effective communication:

"For me, my main concern was to make sure the staff was OK: rounding on them, checking on them, following up."

Vivian, Critical Care Unit Director

"During this time, I tried to make myself more present. Be there to answer questions, all that kind of stuff."

Symone, Education Coordinator for NICU

"I tend to be pretty direct and kind of straight to the point... during Covid, it was really important for me to kind of push that back and take intentional time to sit and inquire. 'How are you doing? How are you taking care of yourself? Have you taken some time off? What are you doing? Then, modeling that in myself, being willing to say, 'I'm really exhausted,' or, 'This is hard for all of us,' and giving people the space to talk about that every day."

Tanja, Unit Director Labor and Delivery

PROMOTE ACTION

"Action is a great restorer and builder of confidence. Inaction is not only the result, but the cause, of fear."
–Norman Vincent Peale, minister and author

The CDC guides that giving people meaningful things to do calms anxiety, helps restore order, and promotes some sense of control. While it would seem that there would be no shortage of tasks for those in healthcare during the pandemic, there was in fact great disparity between departments as routine, preventive, elective, and outpatient clinics closed during the at-home phases, and surges were experienced by intensive care units and emergency departments. These acute units were short-staffed and ill-supplied. New care procedures were being developed for these while other staff were being floated or called off. The huddles previously discussed as important vehicles for the communication of information also allowed for decision-making, delegation of tasks, and evaluation of progress, all important aspects in promoting action:

"Now we huddle Monday, Wednesday, and Friday, and the first thing we do is we go over the Covid situation. We go over any work related to Covid, that takes priority, and then we run through what's our plan for the next day. Everybody has an opportunity to say, 'I'm good to go,' or we have a dashboard that shows all green if they're good to go. Or they may have a red on their dashboard. The red is either related to staffing or information, methods, or workload. If they have a red, then we can call it out. So, it's helped me to understand what the day-to-day work is to be done and helps me understand what problems or barriers they're having, and we can solve them as a team. That's probably been the biggest change, how we communicate and how we prioritize our work. We're doing it as a group three times a week."

Andrew, Chief Quality Officer in Nursing

No one-size-fits-all manner or message of communication would work given the complexity of tasks, but at each turn, the inspiring leader sought to engage their staff and focus on what they could bring to the table. Repeatedly, we heard how our leaders strove to build confidence as they gently pushed their staff to take action and to focus anxieties on overcoming obstacles and developing creative solutions. A crisis situation requires leadership from staff as well as the titled leaders, and an effective leader is able to accept the important contributions staff can bring to the table as they struggle through the nuances of being the front-line managers of care, handling issues and serving to not just disseminate information further down but also convey it back up the chain of command.

> "Communication was so important. The more we communicated and people understood it, the more engaged they were, and they could use it in applicable situations beyond our current crisis . . . and I think that's going to be phenomenal for our organization."
>
> Sharma, Director of Nursing Leadership

> "With Covid, all of a sudden our clinical nurses were making the lead professional governance decisions. That's what professional governance is about: The clinical nurses make the decisions, and the administrators help roll it out to make sure we're all doing what is best for the clinical nurses and clinicians."
>
> Carson, Vice President of Nursing Practice and Education

SHOW RESPECT

"I motivate players through communication, being honest with them, having them respect and appreciate your ability and your help."
—**Tommy Lasorda, baseball player/manager**

Effective communication works best when it reflects appreciation for the contribution of others and the role they share with each other in the process of problem resolution and solution-seeking. This respectful context provides the foundation for considerate interaction, mutual understanding, and collective commitment.

Respectful communication is central to crisis communication when people feel particularly vulnerable. In many ways, returning to the basics of therapeutic communication helps to display respect and promote cooperation and rapport. Sharma, Director of Nursing Leadership, said:

> "Employing active listening, clarifying questions or statements, was critical to developing mutual purpose and sorting through the informational overload that we, as a nation, were receiving."
>
> Sharma, Director of Nursing Leadership

She went on to another facet of demonstrating respect for the receiver in caring for others holistically:

> "When people are feeling particularly overwhelmed, it can be very important to try and prioritize what is necessary, where the starting point is, and what do we need to do with this information to move forward."
>
> Sharma, Director of Nursing Leadership

Central to having this empathy—being available, present, respectful, and vulnerable with staff—was having a culture of trust as the foundation within the organization prior to the crisis. While novel approaches for the delivery of information were often employed, these were built on a depth of mutual respect and credibility.

Sadly, we heard stories from nursing leaders who did not have trust in their administration prior to Covid-19. Sidney was a nurse manager in an outpatient setting for a Federally Qualified Health Center in the Atlanta metro area and struggled with the communication of critical information, lack of PPE, and a sense that nursing staff were more dispensable than physicians and therefore should be put at more risk. She related a story of a patient presenting to the clinic with Covid symptoms who had been with family members who had their Covid-positive status confirmed. Sadly, the medical staff refused to see the patient, and the nurse manager was called to assess him to determine if he should be sent to the hospital.

"So, I went in there and the patient had his mask on. He was looking at his phone, and the room was dark. I'll never forget it because they didn't have the light on, and I wondered, 'Why isn't the light on?' I went in there and asked him questions. He wasn't feeling well. He had a low-grade temp, 99.8 or something like that. He had the cough, but he didn't cough while I was in there. And I just had the facial mask on. I did not have the N95 because they wouldn't let us wear it, so I stepped out. I was so mad. He ended up in the hospital Friday night, in ICU in the Covid area."

Sidney, Federally Qualified Health Center Nursing Director

Clearly, all healthcare organizations were experiencing struggles with obtaining PPE and were challenged to provide optimal care in a world of unknowns at the beginning of the pandemic. In that first month, there was concern that hospitals would run out of N95 masks, and thus supplies were taken from outpatient settings. Those working inpatient with Covid patients were cleaning and reusing their N95s. But what Sidney describes is a culture in which the nurses felt unvalued, disrespected, and dispensable. She was called to see a patient that no other member of the team would see. She felt she was put into a position exposing her to a life-threatening illness. Lack of respect for her role as a valued, critical team member ultimately led to her resignation, a casualty of the Covid-19 pandemic.

THE IMPORTANCE OF REASSURANCE AND TRANSPARENCY

Communication is no more critical in a crisis than it is in any other time. However, the trajectory and focus of communication become more short-term, immediate, and real-time. Because everyone's attention is narrowed and emotions are heightened, the imminence of personal communication accelerates. People need to know what's happening now. They also need to know that those in charge are not overtaken by reaction, impotence, or the critical circumstances. The information that needs to be shared in short order operates at a level of personal safety with the assurance that the attention of the leader will reflect people's concerns and circumstances (Albert et al., 2022).

Communicate essential information quickly and effectively. There is a hierarchy of information that needs to be shared in a crisis. First-line information should be precise, clear, brief, incisive, and relevant. People need to know that those in charge are using the levers of their power and position first to address the crisis and second to communicate the nature of the crisis, its impact and circumstances, and its relationship to the people in the organization. The first reaction of individuals to crisis is, "How does it impact me?" Leaders should understand this level of personalization, and the needs of individuals must be assured, encouraged, and supported. Information sharing at this stage should focus on what is happening, its impact on the organization and its people, the exploration of leaders to dig deeper into the causative factors, and some initial positive responses that leaders are undertaking with suggestions of how those receiving the information might also act.

Share information about what is not known as transparently as what is known. Crisis is a dynamic and, as this chapter indicates, is always shifting and changing in ways that are not predictable and certain. While it is important to share known information about a crisis as soon as possible, it is also important to indicate to staff and others that the trajectory of a crisis is unpredictable and uncertain and that circumstances may quickly shift and change. The context for sharing what is not known about a crisis should help encourage staff through use of language that demonstrates vigilance, access, openness, and availability to respond to the unpredictable vagaries embedded in the processes and activities associated with the crisis. Also, information shared earlier in a crisis may be diametrically changed given better information, more adequate tools of response, and/or new knowledge and experience, including the products of insight and innovation. This radical shift in what is known can often create uncertainty and disequilibrium in people. Leaders, in this case, need to be alert to this reality and continue to remind people of the impact of new insight, knowledge, and responses different from those attempted earlier in the crisis experience.

Affirm confidence in leadership. As noted in a variety of other chapters in this book, leadership competence and confidence are important to teams in confronting and managing crisis roles and experiences. Leaders must demonstrate a consistency and calmness in the face of the "noise" embedded in every crisis moment, circumstance, and situation. A sense of personal steadiness in the face of the intensity and chaos of crisis makes engagement and management of intense crisis events feel possible. This leadership steadiness and confidence create a sense of calm and trust that translates into the capacity to respond and the ability to address the related concerns positively and with a sense of hope and progress.

REIMAGINING COMMUNICATION

The amount and means of communicating vital information changed drastically during the pandemic. The virus itself necessitated alterations in meetings from in-person to virtual whenever possible to limit virus transmission. Given the nature of exponential learning about the novel virus and delivery of care, protocols were constantly changing, and the communication of such was vital to organization reaction and adaptation. Town Hall sessions were held in order to hear from the staff; tiered huddles became vital to solving unit to hospital-wide issues; podcasts were found to be more acceptable to staff than multiple emails; and playbooks were written to adapt information and standardize across multiple facilities and clinics. Throughout all modes and forms of communication, leaders commented on the overload and the need to sort out the various communiques. Leaders provided insights into this problem and how it was managed with various modes of communication:

> "[We were] hosting Zoom meetings where people could just come and have an open forum to talk. We held open forums and Town Halls [for] staff to just come and talk or ask questions. You know, that was twofold, right? We want to get information out to you. But we also want feedback from you, or you to share your thoughts and concerns with us . . . [Leadership hosted] little coffee chats in the main lobby as folks come in. No agenda, just have a cup of coffee and a doughnut. And we're here to greet you to support you to say, 'Good morning' . . . in itself that was helpful for them to see . . . we're all in this together."
>
> Kathy, Chief Nursing Officer

"There was no topic off limits at those command center huddles. They were well-organized, well-structured, and they had an agenda. But if somebody needed to bring something up as a question, it was given the time it deserved to get answered or figure out the next steps. The huddles that we used as part of our Lean and Power Process that we had started probably about a year and a half ago, before the pandemic, really helped us with that."

Andrew, Chief Quality Officer in Nursing

"The podcast is a weekly thing that we send to the staff so we have communication on a daily basis. A lot of times it's hard to rely on people getting to communication that is sent via email. So many times we communicate a lot with our charge nurses as well, for shifts that we are not here for, and we ask them to pass on to the next shift as well."

Vivian, Critical Care Unit Director

"All of the hospitals were initially charged with doing a playbook so that we could have a record of all protocol decisions and documentation. It was like I was rewriting the Bible. We got it all online and had to often rewrite and update components every other day, but it gave us a standard place to house all treatment, protocol, and care decisions . . . so that everyone had access to these standardizations and decisions of practice."

Michelle, Innovation and Advancement Coordinator

Summing up the various modes of communication, one unit director acknowledged all modes but valued the repetition and face-to-face communication as the most influential:

"We have a daily huddle in my department. That was the primary means of communication. It's different people each day, but I put on my calendar to attend all those huddles. For my night shift folks, I had some meetings, and then I'd also call in while they were there and talk to them and go through the same information and answer any questions. It was really just a lot of repetition. People weren't really checking their emails a lot; some information you didn't even want to put in writing because it was going to change so quickly. So really, it was mostly the huddle communication that kept everybody on top of what was going on. We posted things in the office, too. They did give us like a playbook that they would update and that always had the most recent information in it. So, we have that available, but mostly just talking over and over and over again."

Tanja, Unit Director Labor and Delivery

One of the more challenging aspects of the pandemic was communication with family. In the early phases and then with the surges, family members who had once been so central to care delivery were now shut out from the facilities. Patients were dropped off at hospitals by loved ones for necessary surgeries or Covid symptoms with the very real possibility that this could be the last time they would be hugged. For easily the past 20 years, we have as a system committed to including family and providing patient-centered care, realizing better outcomes, less falls, and other complications by having family members engaged in care. Now, by virtue of attempting to limit exposure, patients were isolated and families felt disconnected from their hospitalized family member.

> "We had to identify ways to communicate with the families of the Covid patients... People are desperate about their loved ones: 'What's going on? Why can I not be there?' And we have to change how we communicate with families. So, we adapted some technology to do that."
>
> Vivian, Critical Care Unit Director

Unit directors reported facilitating Skype calls with family members, and staff were using their personal cell phones to allow family to speak with their patients. Daily calls between the medical staff and a family representative were instituted to keep the family informed of the patient's progress.

KEY TAKEAWAYS

Communications must be accurate and complete for decisions to be made, and it is equally as important for the rest of the organization to be provided with complete and acute information. During a crisis, Prewitt et al. (2011) warned that "Information distribution and distortion is likely to place the organization at an even greater disadvantage" (p. 61) than that imposed by just the crisis. Poor crisis communication surrounding the crisis can destroy the response efforts and even the long-term viability of the organization. Information from the top down is important to frame the story and promptly mitigate misinformation. While a high priority must be placed on disseminating information down, an equal amount of attention must be placed on assuring reception with understanding and rapid elevation of any concerns or fallout. Information must be communicated rapidly, honestly, and transparently, in a forthright manner. It is important to let the organization know that you do not know all the facts but then tell them what you do know. It is also crucial that as information becomes available it is communicated to all to ensure that the right steps are being taken.

ADDITIONAL READING ABOUT CRISIS COMMUNICATION

Civelek, M. E., Çemberci, M., & Eralp, N. E. (2016). The role of social media in crisis communication and crisis management. *International Journal of Research in Business & Social Science, 5*(3), 111–120.

Eldridge, C. C., Hampton, D., & Marfell, J. (2020). Communication during crisis. *Nursing Management, 51*(8), 50–53. https://doi.org/10.1097/01.NUMA.0000688976.29383.dc

Jankelová, N., & Joniaková, Z. (2021). Communication skills and transformational leadership style of first-line nurse managers in relation to job satisfaction of nurses and moderators of this relationship. *Healthcare, 9*(3), 346. https://doi.org/10.3390/healthcare9030346

Liu, B., Iles, I. A., & Herovic, E. (2020). Leadership under fire: How governments manage crisis communication. *Communication Studies, 71*(1), 1–20. https://doi.org/10.1080/10510974.2019.1683593

Simonovich, S. D., Spurlark, R. S., Badowski, D., Krawczyk, S., Soco, C., Ponder, T. N., Rhyner, D., Waid, R., Aquino, E., Lattner, C., Wiesemann, L. M., Webber-Ritchey, K., Li, S., & Tariman, J. D. (2021). Examining effective communication in nursing practice during COVID-19: A large-scale qualitative study. *International Nursing Review, 68*(4), 512–523. https://doi.org/10.1111/inr.12690

REFLECTIVE EXERCISES

6.1 → COMMUNICATION EFFECTIVENESS SELF-ASSESSMENT

Think back to a time when you needed to communicate to others as a leader during a crisis. Complete the following flowchart with what needed to be communicated, why this communication was necessary, how the communication occurred, and the feedback you received or further questions or concerns that were raised as a result of this dialogue.

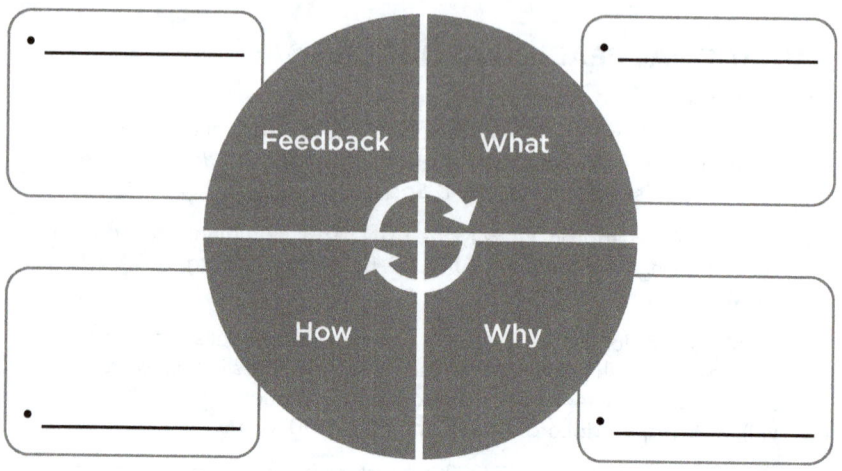

On a scale of 1–10, how would you rate this crisis communication? What could you have done better?

6.2 → CREATE A COMMUNICATION PLAN

List the individual steps you would take to organize a briefing in which you had to present a completely new protocol that needs to be implemented immediately. Consider who needs to be heard from, what evidence is needed, what planning, and who should be involved with communicating the idea further.

6.3 → COMMUNICATION GONE WRONG

Describe a time you had to relay bad news to a client or colleague. How did you assure you communicated with respect?

REFERENCES

Albert, N., Pappas, S., Porter-O'Grady, T., & Malloch, K. (2022). *Quantum leadership*. Jones & Bartlett Learning.

Centers for Disease Control and Prevention. (2018). *CDC's Crisis and Emergency Risk Communication (CERC) manual.* https://emergency.cdc.gov/cerc/manual/index.asp

Oxford English Dictionary. (2021). In *Oxford English Dictionary Online.* https://www-oed-com.

Pagano, P., & Pagano, C. L. (2017). *Health communication for health care professionals: An applied approach.* Springer Publishing Company.

Parvanta, C., & Bass, S. (2020). *Health communication: Strategies for a new era.* Jones & Bartlett.

Prewitt, J. E., Weil, R. S., & McClure, A. Q. (2011). Crisis leadership—An organizational opportunity. *Australian Journal of Business and Management Research*, 1(6), 60–74.

Roosevelt, F. D. (1941). Speech by Franklin D. Roosevelt, New York [Transcript]. https://www.loc.gov/item/afccal000483/

"Alone we can do so little; together we can do so much."
—Helen Keller

7

Teamwork and Collaboration

A nursing leader both collaborates with others and leads teams. At times, these can be synonymous tasks—both teamwork and collaboration involve a group of people working together to complete a shared goal—but subtle differences exist.

W. Edwards Deming, the father of productivity, accountability, and quality, advocated that teamwork was an essential component for business success. In his key principles to managers for transforming business effectiveness, first presented in his book *Out of the Crisis*, Deming's 14th and final principle contended that everybody in the company must work to accomplish transformation. Essentially, he argued that transformation "is everybody's job" (Deming, 2018, p. 397). So, was Deming

> **WE ASKED NURSE LEADERS**
> → Who did you trust to work with you during this crisis?
> → Who supported you in the organization?
> → What partnerships did you develop among other groups within the organization?
> → What other departments have you been working closely with, and how have these relationships changed through the crisis?
> → What were unexpected collaborations and partnerships that developed?

arguing for teamwork to collectively produce the transformation or collaboration? These principles have been widely applied over multiple different types of business, from manufacturing to aviation to healthcare. However, a deep dive into the etymology and linguistics reveals key differences in jargon and intent.

COLLABORATION AND TEAMWORK: CLARIFYING CONCEPTS

The Oxford English Dictionary (OED) defines teamwork as "the action or fact of working together effectively or cohesively; successful collaboration or cooperation by a team of people" (OED, n.d.). This term harkens back to the early 1800s when the term was associated with a team of horses or draught animals ploughing, hauling, or helping with farm work (Brooke, 1800). In teamwork, the individual efforts of all team members are combined to achieve a goal. Teamwork is usually overseen by a team leader, and tasks are individually delegated to members on the team to complete to ultimately contribute to the goal.

The OED defines collaboration as "united labour, co-operation; esp. in literary, artistic, or scientific work" but also has a secondary meaning from World War II, when collaboration had a negative connotation indicating "traitorous cooperation with the enemy" (OED, 2018). Collaboration is a higher level of cooperation where people work collaboratively to complete a project collectively. Those collaborating work together as equals, usually without a leader, to come up with ideas or make decisions together to complete a goal. A collaborative group is self-managed, with various members stepping up to lead aspects of the project, but all equally sharing in formulating the direction and completing the tasks necessary to achieve the team objective.

Collaborative group formation is necessary when the objective requires more complex thinking and strategizing, particularly when outcomes depend on the actions of several departments or professionals. These collaborations may be permanent structures or temporary depending on this need and mission. We suggest that if collaborations between professionals can relate and strategize using interdisciplinary or transdisciplinary collaboration, results can be compounded. This type of powerful collaboration requires everyone in the group to employ communication and leadership savvy as there may not be one specific leader or coach, and leadership may rotate because all professionals on this team are capable.

Teamwork combines the individual efforts of all members to achieve a goal under the direction of a leader. Think of a Major League baseball team under the direction of a coach. All team members can hit, throw, catch, and run. Worse comes to worst, a first baseman can likely play outfield if the coach directed him to. Clearly, individual players have things they are better at and have distinct roles from pitching to hitting to fielding. They follow directions and combine their individual skills to win the game. In baseball, as with most teams, an individual player does not take a turn as the coach or challenge the coach when they decide to change the batting order or bring in a relief pitcher. With a collaborative group, the members of the group should collectively analyze the problem, jointly decide the plan, and share leadership.

COORDINATING COLLABORATION DURING CRISIS: THE INCIDENT COMMAND SYSTEM

As we have discussed throughout this book, the organizational approach to leadership of a healthcare entity will need to change during a crisis. The Incident Command System (ICS) is a standardized approach to the command, control, and coordination of leadership responses providing a standardized hierarchy that allows a coordinated response from multiple collaborating teams (US Department of Transportation, Federal Highway Administration, n.d.). Initially developed to address problems of inter-agency responses to wildfires in California and Arizona, ICS has been tested by more than 30 years of emergency and non-emergency applications and is a central component of the National Incident Management System (NIMS; Irwin, 1989). Because all levels of government (such as the Federal Emergency Management Agency [FEMA]) and many private critical organizations (including all Medicare and Joint Commission hospitals) are required to have emergency response plans that include an established ICS, most have adopted a standard management hierarchy and procedures for managing crisis incidents of any size.

The ICS structure is successful because it:

- Is interdisciplinary in nature
- Utilizes a common language that is used across disciplines
- Outlines clear lines of communication
- Allows for flexibility to cope with various types and complexities of incidents

ICS consists of a hierarchy of roles to launch pre-established procedures for the temporary management of funds, personnel, facilities, equipment, and communications. Leadership personnel are pre-identified and trained on the structure and various roles (Werman et al., 2014).

As discussed in Chapter 5, certain leadership traits may be useful for the determination of leadership roles in an ICS incident. It may well be that during a crisis, the CEO is not the Incident Commander because another senior leadership person has a greater depth of understanding of the particular situation or a leadership style that is more befitting Incident Commander than the CEO. Similarly, in a protracted situation, leadership roles will need to be rotated between members to prevent both physical and psychological fatigue.

INCIDENT COMMAND SYSTEM GUIDE AND FEMA TRAININGS

The third edition of the NIMS, published in 2017 by FEMA, is a free printable book that provides a comprehensive guide for how government, nongovernmental organizations, and the private sector work together to prevent, protect against, mitigate, respond to, and recover from incidents. It is available at https://www.fema.gov/sites/default/files/2020-07/fema_nims_doctrine-2017.pdf.

An updated list of available FEMA-associated trainings and certifications for incident command and emergency response are available at https://www.fema.gov/emergency-managers/national-preparedness/training#individuals or through your state Emergency Management Agency. Online and community trainings are frequently offered and are essential for any personnel that would assume a leadership role in emergency preparedness, incident response, or the Hospital Command Center (Hospital Emergency Operations Center).

Specific courses should include:
- → ICS 100: Basics of ICS
- → ICS 200: Applying ICS to Healthcare Organizations
- → IS 700: Introduction to NIMS

Carson, Vice President of Nursing Practice and Education, described the ICS structure, roles, and responsibilities within their healthcare system:

> "We have an ICC, our Incident Command Council Committee, that meets. We call them Team Six: the CEO, CO, Chief Executive Nurse. They are the ones with the final say. But [the decision-making is] still not [up to] an individual on those teams; they come to consensus as a group. Then there are all these subgroups around the health system. We are meeting daily to build reports, to build proposals, to build research, to help us make the best decisions we can make at the time. For example, I'm in the process of working with a team called clinical operations to help set up visitation policies to determine how we can bring family members back in the hospital to be with the patient."
>
> Carson, Vice President of Nursing Practice and Education

FOUNDATIONAL PRINCIPLES FOR COLLABORATION

As with many leadership tenets, many have attempted to define the essential components of effective collaboration. We will explore some previously published models and ideas related to collaboration before sharing from our research the themes that arose most strongly during our interviews.

HACKMAN'S TEAM COACHING MODEL

The basics of team collaboration and effectiveness were identified by J. Richard Hackman, a pioneer in the field of organizational behavior, who began studying teams in the 1970s. He postulated after more than 40 years of research that there are certain conditions necessary for team success, as outlined in Figure 7.1.

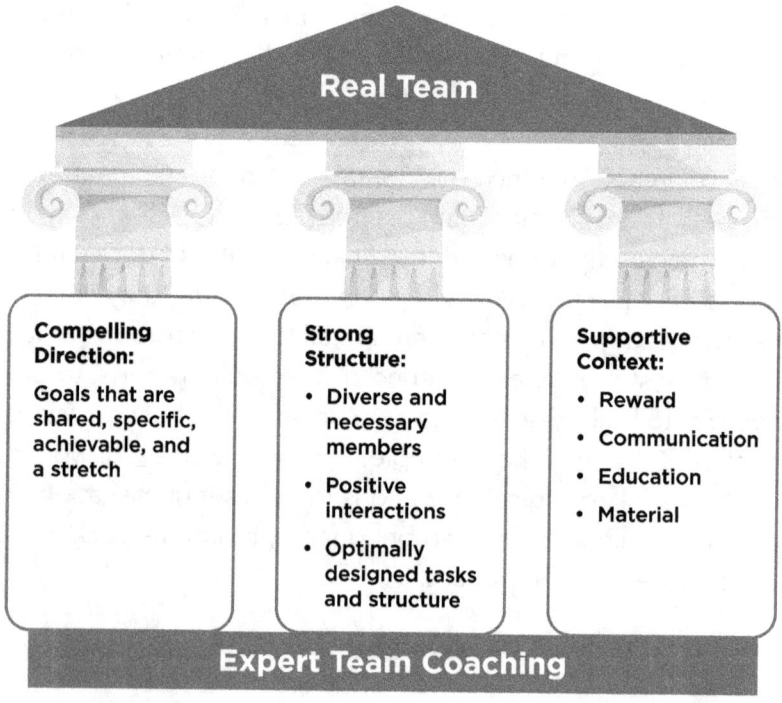

FIGURE 7.1 Hackman's Team Coaching Model.

The first component is that a team must be established with legitimacy and stability of group membership over time. The three pillars then support the team:

- The first pillar is a compelling direction for the work, which encompasses having goals that are shared, specific, achievable, and have consequences. Goals should cause teams to stretch and work to achieve a specific goal.

- The second pillar is for a strong, enabling structure comprised of only necessary members who are diverse in specialty, age, background, and experience. With diversity comes creativity. The positivity and structure of processes and roles should be stressed.
- Supportive components comprise the third pillar in the form of reward, communication, education, and material resources and support.

Undergirding all three pillars is knowledgeable and expert coaching and leadership of the teams.

AGBANYIM'S PRINCIPLES OF COLLABORATION

In his well-received general leadership book, J. Ibeh Agbanyim similarly outlined five principles of collaboration (2015):

1. Trust
2. Respect
3. Willingness
4. Empowerment
5. Effective communication

These principles have been recognized as applicable across business, personal, and intimate relationships, fostering individual and professional success.

AHRQ MODEL OF COLLABORATION

Specific to healthcare, the Agency for Healthcare Research and Quality (AHRQ) defined collaboration as "disciplines working together, sharing responsibility for problem-solving, and making decisions to formulate and deliver care" (Hughes, 2008, p. 272). Similar to Agbanyim, this AHRQ publication stressed trust, respect, and collaboration as essential components of effective teams.

OUR THEMATIC INTERVIEWS

As we analyzed our interviews, the major themes that emerged were a commitment to the team, trust, communication, clear definition of roles and responsibilities, a commitment to inclusion, and positive leadership, motivation, and mentoring. To best visualize and validate these themes, we aligned them with the foundational constructs put forth by the previous authorities in Table 7.1.

TABLE 7.1 Comparison of Collaboration Models

	J. Richard Hackman's 5 Conditions	J. Ibeh Agbanyim Principles of Collaboration	AHRQ	Thematic Interviews
Focus	Working team			Commitment to team
Directionality	Compelling direction; goals			Shared vision
Characteristics	Strong structure: diversity and operational structure	Trust; respect; willingness	Trust; respect	Trust; clear definition of roles and responsibilities
Outcomes	Supportive components: reward, communication, educational, and material resources and support	Effective communication	Collaboration	Communication
Process	Team coaching	Empowerment		Positive leadership, motivation, and mentoring

COMMITMENT TO A SHARED MISSION

In our interviews, we learned from the nurse leaders that they felt collaboration was best when there was an acknowledged commitment to the mission of the team regardless of position or role. Repeatedly, we heard from high-ranking leaders that there was no task beneath them, no ball that was tossed and allowed to fall because another person didn't run to catch it. Members of the team—whether it be the formal Incident Command System for a large hospital system, a Clinical Operations Team, or a Surgical Services Oversight Team making decisions for which surgeries should be postponed—must have: 1) a commitment to the team's objectives, and 2) a commitment to seeing the objectives completed regardless of the demands, assigned and unassigned roles, and tasks. It is with this commitment that teamwork becomes true collaboration.

Kimberly, Nurse Anesthetist and Nursing Faculty, spoke considerably about the teamwork undertaken by the anesthesia department at her large healthcare system, stressing that while the surgical and anesthesia team she served on was quite diverse with representative members from anesthetists, anesthesiologists, nurses, and surgeons, they were united in the team's objectives to limit the transmission of Covid and keep all staff safe. This meant making some hard choices, as a team, regarding the provision of CPR, how patients were intubated, the choice of anesthesia, and determining which patients met criteria they collaboratively created for urgent surgery:

"We started meeting with the surgical services team every week, and we discussed several things. First of all, as anesthesia providers we decided we had to change our anesthetics. Everybody had to do the same anesthetic, the same way, no matter what. It didn't matter what the case was, there was to be only one approach. That was a very protective approach for our providers; even if the surgeon was doing a case that was challenging, we (the anesthesia team) were going to still protect ourselves to the full extent that we could in terms of PPE and the way we took care of the patient. Another approach is we collaborated with surgical services on the cases that were non-emergent versus emergent. And we had surgeons . . . a surgical committee or the Chief of Surgery at our hospital, who, along with an anesthesiologist, had to review every single case that got done."

Kimberly, Nurse Anesthetist and Nursing Faculty

She went on to describe that there were times that surgeons (not on the oversight team) did not want to postpone elective surgeries or attempted to circumvent the system developed. In these instances, the leaders of this Surgical Services Oversight Team were called upon to assist the wayward surgeon to understand the mission of the team. It was the collaboration that overrode most aspects of usual operation in this time of crisis.

A commitment to the team's objectives can mean that there needs to be singularity in purpose and requires strength of the team leadership to stay focused on this objective. Too often, collaboration can get sidetracked by adding on subtasks; they may seem important to some, but they divert attention from collaborating on solving the primary issue. An excellent example of this was articulated by Andrew, Chief Quality Officer in Nursing, who needed to immediately remove any discussions about the cost of a given solution as it distracted from exploring all possibilities:

"To figure out the scope of those things and what were the deadlines around doing it? Now, how critical were they? What was the scope of what we were supposed to do versus what was out of bounds for us to do? And we had to work quickly; in the Intermediate Care Unit, our job was to define what the criteria guidelines' trigger points and processes are for setting up an intermediate care unit. But we're not tackling anything with regards to resources or funding. That was outside of our wheelhouse. We made those statements very clear upfront and said these things are off the table. We don't discuss those (funding), even though we had challenges with people wanting to discuss them."

Andrew, Chief Quality Officer in Nursing

Membership on a team could be assigned or they may volunteer, as Andrew went on to describe:

"The Chief Nursing Executive said, 'Hey, can you do this, and can you do it with this person?' It was a mix of being assigned, and a mix of being willing and being capable of taking a team and putting them through a formal approach to assessing a problem. Collaborating on what potential solutions could be and then defining our options to the leadership team and making the final decision. I think we were more nimble than we usually were, and it was certainly a mix of assignment and volunteering."

Andrew, Chief Quality Officer in Nursing

Sometimes teams developed organically, such as Kimberly's:

"So, the weekend of . . . of March 6th, 7th, and 8th I had two or three people call me, inquiring about what is happening: 'We haven't heard anything from our leadership. We haven't heard anything from the hospital. It sounds like this is coming . . . what are we doing?' I called the chief of our group, and he told me that the hospital had put together this team, and they were meeting, and we had an infectious disease specialist on board, and so it was really that weekend where everybody really got concerned and formed a team."

Kimberly, Nurse Anesthetist and Nursing Faculty

TRUST

"Collaboration flourishes in an atmosphere where there is a high level of trust among the disciplines" (Akhavain et al., 1999, p. 2). Trust is a crucial antecedent for collaboration and is necessary to allow team members to readily assume accountability and responsibility, understanding that trust and respect for individual perspectives are part of the team's culture (Pike et al., 1993).

Team members must trust that they are valued and are committed to the mission; trust that they are vested in the mission's success such that they will contribute their best; trust within members to step up to do anything necessary (nothing is beneath them); and trust that team members essentially have the backs of others on the team. The element of trust that was surprising was how the leaders of these teams used the word "trust" in allowing others on the teams to lead and trusting the decisions made by subordinates. Trust on a team surpasses usual hierarchy and allows for all members on that team to have a voice, contribution, and sometimes even support the leader of the team:

"That's the kind of leadership that I aspire to and the leadership that I was trying to practice and build before Covid: to trust my team. I've got an amazing team to know that they're more connected with the nurses we work with, and I am too."

Carson, Vice President of Nursing Practice and Education

The effective leader builds trust within their team through trusting his team. We observed this in talking with Andrew:

"I don't see leadership as being someone who makes all the decisions. I try to make fewer decisions. I tried to guide people into defining what the goals are, and then setting resources in place to be able to get to those goals. Leadership to me is being willing to listen, it's being willing to kind of step outside of my own ego and wanting to get things done. Listening to what's possible, what we need to do, what the barriers are, what the opportunities and promises are, and then helping people to work towards those goals."

Andrew, Chief Quality Officer in Nursing

Another aspect to effective teams is that leaders can trust that the necessary work will continue even when they are pulled away. During the pandemic, leaders were tapped to wear many hats and pulled away from usual operations that still had to continue. Andrew discussed how trust in his usual operations team was essential and reassuring:

"Luckily, I have a wonderful team that I can trust, a great quality director, and two excellent quality analysts, and they kept that piece going. We still had to do the reporting. We still had our Magnet submissions or quality submissions, all that; we didn't start anything new there. In my informatics team we're still working on largely things like unit, new units, or changing units from med/surg to critical care. Or, IT changes that needed to occur in the electronic medical record around the care of Covid patients. So, I relied heavily on my teams to take care of that work and to keep me updated."

Andrew, Chief Quality Officer in Nursing

Trust, however, is not omnipresent. It waxes and wanes and needs nourishment and sometimes resuscitation as discussed by Carson:

"Trust has been huge, although it is hard at times as we get stressed out. Sometimes trust fizzles, and I've seen that in my team. I've seen that in other teams. It's natural; it's human. You are actively recognizing that you must rebuild and support trust."

Carson, Vice President of Nursing Practice and Education

COMMUNICATION

Effective communication remains the backbone of just about every process we've discussed in this book, and collaborating within a unit-based team, inter-department or interdisciplinary team is no different. Collaboration simply cannot exist without effective communication. In crisis situations, we have recommended formal crisis communication training, as discussed in Chapter 6. Imperative is that lines of communication are established before a crisis so that a base of trust exists to support this communication. Andrew, part of the Incident Command System for his large hospital system, acknowledged:

"Having built into our infrastructure relationships with the CDC and patterns of communication and dialogue . . . helped us to have a mindset to know how to listen to the sciences. In developing our practices, those relationships and lines of open communication were invaluable."

Andrew, Chief Quality Officer in Nursing

Communication is most noteworthy when it is not present, or when it fails to happen effectively. When asked about effective communication between teams, every leader had a story about that botched or disastrous communication exchange. This is one of those situations in which the best example of communication on teams is a contrary example. Carson described not having an effective communication strategy of a new protocol due to the time-sensitive, urgent nature of putting the protocol into place:

"Trying to roll out a new policy to another entity without clear communication, without understanding and bringing teams together, but instead just saying, 'Go and do this,' . . . it didn't work as well. Because a lot of people had questions, and if you have a lot of questions, they are not going to do it."

Carson, Vice President of Nursing Practice and Education

The corollary then is that effective communication is occurring if objectives are being met, decisions are being made, and creativity is abounding.

CLEARLY DEFINED ROLES AND RESPONSIBILITIES

One of the structural elements discussed earlier in this chapter is the ICS and the recommendation to undertake NIMS training. Within this structure are very clear roles, responsibilities, and lines of communication that facilitate, rather than impede, collaboration. A crisis is any situation that overwhelms resources of an organization or system. By the very nature of the event, no single person can solve the issue, yet there is a human tendency for many to want to be involved or solve every aspect of a crisis.

Training in ICS helps the leaders to understand that their assigned specific role is critical and needs their complete attention. No single person can be involved with every decision or aspect of the crisis response, nor should they be. Healthcare response to Covid has been epic and protracted, with multiple permutations and consequences that no one person could have envisioned and no one person or team could solve. The necessity of clearly assigned roles and even clearly defined responsibilities for specific teams was critical. Andrew described this structure and the roles:

"There were several groups that reported out to the Incident Command Center. We have a Clinical Operations Group, and they largely focused on the things that are needed to keep clinical operations stable: staffing, visitation policies, which services continue to be provided in a surge and which services don't. Then there's the Care Model Team, the group that defined how we provided care both for Covid patients and for non-Covid patients. Not necessarily the treatment parameters around those patients but how to safely care for Covid patients. Proper Covid ID policies when someone is a suspected Covid patient, but they don't have a lab result yet. How many patients and what types of patients should get rapid Covid tests versus standard, a referral lab test that may or may not take three or four days to come back? That group's been really wonderful. It's a group of doctors, nurses, administrators, led by epidemiology and infection prevention. All of those groups have been wonderful, and I think it's really been a foray for our system into a higher level of governance and decision-making than perhaps we had before. People have an understanding that within that ability to be quick, there must be some level of system-ness and standardization."

Andrew, Chief Quality Officer in Nursing

COMMITMENT TO INCLUSION OF DIVERSE KNOWLEDGE AND PERSPECTIVES

Inclusion of the right persons and the right disciplines within a team fosters understanding, innovation, risk-taking, and superior outcomes. How disciplines, departments, scientists, and even colleagues interact on a team to meet a common objective has varied depending on the organization. Team sciences started differentiating these research disciplines in the 1990s, adopting the terms intradisciplinary, multidisciplinary, interdisciplinary, and transdisciplinary (Stember, 1991). Spreading to healthcare, many organizations adopted the structure to promote better patient care. Without understanding the subtle differences, these terms have been used interchangeably by many, but they are in fact distinct concepts, as described in a concept analysis done over 20 years ago and aggregated into Table 7.2 (Reilly, 2001).

TABLE 7.2 Disciplinarity Concepts and Attributes

Disciplinarity Concept	Definition	Goals	Key Attributes
Intradisciplinary	Working within a single discipline	Limited to those that can be developed, articulated, and measured by the specific discipline	Same discipline working together as a team May be limited by scope of practice or depth of knowledge
Multidisciplinary	Different disciplines working together, each drawing on their disciplinary knowledge	Develop distinct discipline-specific goals Can set goals for the team that are achieved by specific people with the specific knowledge and training	Clearly defined roles for each team member Each team member functions independently, from their discipline perspective Collaboration on vision, but may result in silos
Interdisciplinary	Integrating knowledge and methods from different disciplines to synthesize approaches/ decisions	Goal setting and visioning is done as a group, collaboratively. Recommendations are a result of group decision-making that may include problem solving beyond an individual's particular knowledge base.	While each team member brings their disciplinary approach, they collaborate on goals and mission that includes all perspectives and may participate in collaborative work that marries actions from one discipline with actions or evaluations from another.

Transdisciplinary	Creating a unity of intellectual frameworks beyond the disciplinary perspectives	Goals and team recommendations are based on the mission or goal at hand, and not on team members' expertise. The ultimate goal is to promote integrated assessment and to develop a unified plan that can be executed by any of the team members.	Research or delivery of care transcends the normal boundaries of a specific field of study, such that individual discipline team members bring expertise, but they freely engage in educating others and sharing tasks that can be performed by anyone acquiring the skill set (within scope of practice limits).

Teams' level of commitment to inclusion can be fostered as the level of disciplinarity increases from intradisciplinary to transdisciplinary. The higher the integration and commitment to inclusion and diversity through the sharing of knowledge and tasks, the argument can be made that outcomes are more creative, timely, and economical. Stember (1991, p. 2) put forth several arguments for higher disciplinarity engagement: "The intellectual argument for interdisciplinary work is that ideas in any field are enriched by theories, concepts, and methods from other fields. Specialization in disciplines and subdisciplines has yielded tremendous gains in knowledge, but specialization is also the fragmentation of mind and subject matter."

While some could argue that transdisciplinary should be a goal for most teams, it is not practical or wise for all teams in all situations. The degree of cross integration is not the objective, but the simple integration of disciplines and inclusion of viewpoints previously not considered should be the goal for teamwork. This applies to leadership during routine operations, but especially in times of crisis. Consider Amber, Nurse Entrepreneur and Professor, expressing the need to not just listen to diverse viewpoints but facilitate their development as a point of leadership:

"A leader with vision will take the time to understand the best way to implement that plan of creating, whatever it is, whatever your vision is, but not alone. So much of it is building a team. . . I think that there's an instinct in finding the right people, just knowing that they'd be a great person to be on your team. With that comes the ability to really listen, to take the time to listen and understand people, to make that connection with them. So, it gets back to that connection. If I'm interviewing someone to be a member of the team, I need to be open to that moment with that individual, pulling those folks together to get their expertise, being receptive and open."

Amber, Nurse Entrepreneur and Associate Professor

Time and again, we heard the need to have the right people with diverse viewpoints on the team:

"It's kind of an all-hands-on-deck situation and it really wasn't necessarily based on anyone's title or position; it was based on our willingness to reach out to people who we thought could help drive requirements and process the policy, and then quickly lead a team to do it."

Andrew, Chief Quality Officer in Nursing

This willingness to include diverse specialties, roles, and personalities on the teams with a focused objective allowed for heightened productivity:

"It was really just everybody coming together, and it was impressive how quickly, not only those things came through, but how quickly other things came through with people leading them that may not have traditionally led."

Tanja, Unit Director Labor and Delivery

The more inclusive and open teams are to higher levels of disciplinarity, the more blended roles become as members share knowledge and tasks. A transdisciplinary approach is good for a working team with not just thought but action outcomes that must operationalize new processes themselves. In a truly transdisciplinary team, members are secure in their role and understand that individual contributions are facilitating positive outcomes. Outside of discipline-specific scope of practice limitations, tasks are completed by any team member with the requisite knowledge. All participate in both thought tasks and scut work. Although the unique contributions of each discipline should be valued, role, turf, and status are not elements of a transdisciplinary teams (Akhavain et al., 1999; Lamorey & Ryan, 1998).

POSITIVE LEADERSHIP, MOTIVATION, AND MENTORING

This chapter has focused primarily on collaboration from the stance of a team member. But effective teams must have the appropriate leadership, motivation, and mentoring to produce. Ronald Reagan, the 40th President of the United States, supported that a great leader is one who understands how to motivate and lead a team: "The greatest leader is not necessarily the one who does the greatest things. He is the one that gets people to do the greatest things" (Burr, 2018). In our discussions with the leadership mentors we interviewed, several insights into team leadership were articulated by the most productive leaders.

Leaders must know their team. From Rebecca, Director of Nursing Education at a large hospital system, we learned:

> "I think a leader really recognizes their team, their strengths, what motivates them. I think that being a good leader is knowing that you don't have to know everything or do everything. But recognizing what is in your team."
>
> Rebecca, Director of Nursing Education

Similarly, valuing and trusting the team are critical actions to demonstrate. As Carson, Vice President of Nursing Practice and Education, described, the best way to lead team members was to allow them to direct policies and actions.

> "I trust my team. I've got an amazing team . . . so to trust, build support, and let them lead and then I make subtle changes which can help change the direction we ship."
>
> Carson, Vice President of Nursing Practice and Education

Have manageable-sized teams such that you can develop relationships with each team member. As Tanja, Unit Director Labor and Delivery, relayed, she felt her small team was much more collegial and productive than teams of larger numbers because:

"I think that I'm able to make more one-on-one connections with them and have more of a personal relationship."

Tanja, Unit Director Labor and Delivery

Consistently encourage and praise your team, every effort, the slightest improvement.

"Leadership to me is being willing to support your team and encourage them to be the best that they can, helping them figure out how to break down goals set for themselves, or the goals that we need for them [to pursue] for the organization."

Andrew, Chief Quality Officer in Nursing

LEADERSHIP PRINCIPLES FROM DALE CARNEGIE'S *HOW TO WIN FRIENDS & INFLUENCE PEOPLE*

While we were analyzing these subthemes, it struck us that these recommendations were as old as theories of relationships and leadership itself. A quick perusal of the bookshelf led us to Dale Carnegie's *How to Win Friends & Influence People*, originally published in 1936. Revised in 1981, this book is a graceful admonition in how to be kind, motivational, and productive. While a new edition was marketed for the digital age in 2011, we recommend finding one of the original 30 million copies and rereading every few years as a timeless classic.

Principle 1: Begin with praise and honest appreciation.

Principle 2: Call attention to people's mistakes indirectly.

Principle 3: Talk about your own mistakes before criticizing the other person.

Principle 4: Ask questions instead of giving direct orders.

Principle 5: Let the other person save face.

Principle 6: Praise the slightest improvement and praise every improvement. Be "hearty in your approbation and lavish in your praise."

Principle 7: Give the other person a fine reputation to live up to.

Principle 8: Use encouragement. Make the fault seem easy to correct.

Principle 9: Make the other person happy about doing.

WORKING WITH TEAMS

No one is born to leadership. Whatever else it is, leadership is a learned skill. As the character of teams change in a post-digital age, it is important that leaders also change and represent in their personal leadership role the capacity to adapt and shift behaviors in keeping with the demand for such shifts. The practice environment will always be changing and shifting in keeping with transformations in technology, science, medicine, social understanding, and nursing practice.

Also true is the reality that nurse leaders will always be working with teams. The character and circumstances influencing these teams will also shift as the roles and demands of team members shift in order to maintain relevance in addressing current issues. This requires a deeper and more complex understanding of the leader's role, especially its patterns and expressions. This person leads teams today that are more knowledgeable, broad-based, and interdependent. In a fast-paced and continuously emerging complex system, a team leader may need to be more directive and discursive during times of crisis, and at other times will need to be more engaging, appreciative, and collateral. This notion of "relevance" is an important aspect of the team leader's role as considered in professional work environments.

ESSENTIAL COMPONENTS OF NURSING TEAM LEADERSHIP

Nursing requires an intense level of colleagueship, collaboration, and collateral decision-making. Furthermore, professional workers desire a greater appreciation and full participation in decisions and processes that affect what they do and how they relate. Current models of professional governance address this understanding of the unique character of professionals and the needs of professional teams. Professional team leadership (nursing professional governance) demonstrates particular characteristics that are important to both the leader of professional teams and professional team members, including encouraging open communication, supporting continued learning, emphasizing accountability, focusing on positive change, and staying connected to the realities of the clinical nurse role (Malloch & Porter-O'Grady, 2022).

ENCOURAGING OPEN COMMUNICATION

Nurses must have space in the work environment that allows for conversation, dialogue, exploration, and consultation between and among professional members while undertaking their practice. The work environment and the relationships which represent it must allow for a higher level of this kind of interaction in order for the outcomes of practice to benefit from the fruits of professional interaction.

SUPPORTING CONTINUED LEARNING

Professionals are always learning. Indeed, their environment presents a landscape of continuous adaptation and adjustment as emerging evidence in practice calls for new levels of understanding, accelerated response to quick changes in knowledge, and new applications driven by new technology and tools of practice.

EMPHASIZING ACCOUNTABILITY

Professionals are driven by accountability not responsibility. While responsibility focuses on action, function, task, and the caliber of that effort, accountability focuses on change, impact, and making a difference. While both are essential in the workplace, for the professional, the ability to have an impact, to make a difference, and to change the trajectory for patients represent the forces that underpin the work of the profession. The nurse improves practice not for its own sake, but instead to influence the health and life of the person the nurse will impact (Porter-O'Grady, 2019).

FOCUSING ON POSITIVE CHANGE

Professionals drive toward a positive impact. Regardless of the outcome or the conditions and circumstances of the patient, the primary professional role of the nurse is to positively influence the factors associated with the patient and their circumstances. Professional goals are driven by the urge for positive change: from sickness to health, enabling adaptation to deficits, maximizing support towards a peaceful death, etc. Nurses require a high level of positive leadership that recognizes the responsive needs of this work and helps sustain the nurse's commitment to it in all circumstances.

STAYING CONNECTED TO THE REALITIES OF THE CLINICAL NURSE ROLE

Because the leader of nurses is generally a nurse, it is important that this leader recognize and empathize with the conditions and circumstances of the clinical nurse's work. Professionals expect from their own a deep comprehension of the motives, urges, and values of the professional nurse and their practice. Professionals expect their leaders to demonstrate knowledge, capacity, and understanding of the character and content of the nursing role and its unique circumstances.

The character and the value of professional nursing is bound up in the content and quality of the journey rather than in any particular event or outcome that might be specifically identified with the role. Understanding the nurse is bound up in comprehending the nature and quality of the practice as nurses work to inform, guide, and facilitate a healing journey generally best led by the patient. It is in this understanding that the exemplars of leadership are best demonstrated. Here it can be understood that the nurse leader appreciates the importance and the value of ownership, engagement, inclusion, collaboration, and colleagueship in the expression of the role, as a member of the profession, linking these characteristics to the exercise of leadership and to their relationship with professional nursing colleagues. Bearing witness to these unique characteristics, the nurse leader does not occupy a vertically delineated position with the professional nursing staff. Instead, the nurse leader, regardless of position, is predominantly collateral, collaborative, partnering, and engaging the professional staff in dialogue, deliberation, decision-making, application, and evaluation of nursing action no matter where it occurs. It is these leadership behaviors which best represent team dynamics in a professional context and most uniquely evidence the team characteristics of the professional nurse (Malloch & Porter-O'Grady, 2022).

KEY TAKEAWAYS

This chapter provided an overview of teamwork and collaboration from a variety of perspectives. Both teamwork and collaboration are necessary during routine times, but that need is heightened during crisis situations. It is important to note that during protracted situations like the pandemic, roles may need to be rotated to fresh leaders to allow for rest and rejuvenation. Additionally, innovative teamwork requires a diverse team composition.

In the next chapter, we will discuss how teamwork and collaboration are integral components in assuring organizational continuity and standardization.

REFLECTIVE EXERCISES

7.1 → EFFECTIVE COLLABORATION AND TEAMWORK

In your experience, what are key foundational constructs for effective teamwork and collaboration? What are barriers you have identified in your practice?

Necessary elements for teamwork and collaboration:

Barriers to effective teamwork and collaboration:

7.2 → INSTILLING MOTIVATION

Using the STARR technique, describe a time where you needed to lead a team with motivation to effect a significant change in practice or care.

What strategies did you employ to motivate your team?

Which elements failed or required revision? How were these revised?

Remember, STARR stands for:

> **Situation:** Describe the challenging situation.
>
> **Task:** Describe the task at hand or target desired.
>
> **Action:** Describe the actions taken and possibly the alternatives available.
>
> **Results:** Describe the outcome of your actions, including the ability to meet your objective.
>
> **Reflection:** This extra "R" aims to present your ability to learn and iterate. What did you learn? What would you do differently, the same, or better next time being posed with a similar situation?

7.3 → LEADERSHIP ROLES COMPATIBLE WITH ICS

Given your knowledge of the ICS, contemplate the various roles within the structure. Identify three leadership roles that you think you would be best able to function within. What strengths would you bring to these roles and what challenges do you suspect you might struggle with?

REFERENCES

Agbanyim, J. I. (2015). *The five principles of collaboration: Applying trust, respect, willingness, empowerment, and effective communication to human relationships*. iUniverse.

Akhavain, P., Amaral, D., Murphy, M., & Nehlingerr, K. C. (1999). Collaborative practice: A nursing perspective of the psychiatric interdisciplinary treatment team. *Holistic Nursing Practice, 13*(2), 1–11.

Brooke, W. (1800). *True causes present distress for provisions: How is the ploughing, the drawing, and all kind of team-work to be performed without horses?* C. Whittingham.

Burr, D. (2018). *Ronald Reagan, quotes and quips*. Chartwell Books.

Carnegie, D. (1981). *How to win friends & influence people* (Revised ed.). Simon & Schuster.

Deming, W. E. (2018). *Out of the crisis* (Reissue). MIT Press.

Hughes, R. G. (2008). *Patient safety and quality: An evidence-based handbook for nurses*. Agency for Healthcare Research and Quality.

Irwin, R. L. (1989). Chapter 7: The Incident Command System (ICS). In E. Auf Der Heide, *Disaster response: Principles of preparation and coordination*. C. V. Mosby Company. https://web.archive.org/web/20080423021922/http:/orgmail2.coe-dmha.org/dr/DisasterResponse.nsf/section/07?opendocument&home=html

Lamorey, S., & Ryan, S. (1998). From contention to implementation: A comparison of team practices and recommended practices across service delivery models. *Infant-Toddler Intervention, 8*(4), 309–331.

Malloch, K., & Porter-O'Grady, T. (2022). *Appreciative leadership: Building sustainable partnerships for health*. Jones & Bartlett Learning.

Oxford English Dictionary. (n.d.). *Teamwork*. In Oxford English Dictionary online. https://www.oed.com/

Oxford English Dictionary. (2018). *Collaboration*. In Oxford English Dictionary online. https://www.oed.com/

Pike, A., McHugh, M., Canney, K., Miller, N., Reilly, P., & Seibert, C. (1993). A new architecture for quality assurance: Nurse-physician collaboration. *Journal of Nursing Care Quality, 7*(3), 1–8

Porter-O'Grady, T. (2019). Principles for sustaining shared/professional governance in nursing. *Nursing Management, 50*(1), 36–41. doi: 10.1097/01.NUMA.0000550448.17375.28

Reilly, C. M. (2001). Transdisciplinary approach: An atypical strategy for improving outcomes in rehabilitation and long-term acute care settings. *Rehabilitation Nursing, 26*(6), 216–220, 244. https://doi.org/10.1002/j.2048-7940.2001.tb01958.x

Stember, M. (1991). Advancing the social sciences through the interdisciplinary enterprise. *The Social Science Journal, 28*(1), 1–14. https://doi.org/10.1016/0362-3319(91)90040-B

US Department of Transportation, Federal Highway Administration. (n.d.). *Glossary: Simplified guide to the Incident Command System for transportation professionals.* https://ops.fhwa.dot.gov/publications/ics_guide/glossary.htm

Werman, H. A., Karren, K., & Mistovich, J. (2014). National Incident Management System: Incident Command System. In A. H. Werman, J. Mistovich, & K. Karren (Eds.), *Prehospital emergency care* (10th ed., p. 1217). Pearson Education.

"Mere change is not growth. Growth is the synthesis of change and continuity, and where there is no continuity there is no growth."
—C. S. Lewis, author

8

Ensuring Continuity and Standardization During Rapid Change

Prior to the pandemic, healthcare organizations and providers addressed organizational continuity by developing emergency response plans, running mock scenario drills, and consulting the leading authorities in preparedness. In the previous 20 years, healthcare professionals had become adept at bringing about change to improve quality, safety, and cost-effectiveness. PDCA (Plan, Do, Check, and Act; see Figure 8.1) had become the mantra of nearly every professional, whether delivering care at the bedside or evaluating data in an office.

WE ASKED NURSE LEADERS

→ What issues did you have with continuity or standardization?

→ What sources/data/information did you use to determine changes in policies and procedures?

→ How did you assure changes were implemented across the system?

→ What were unexpected collaborations and partnerships that developed?

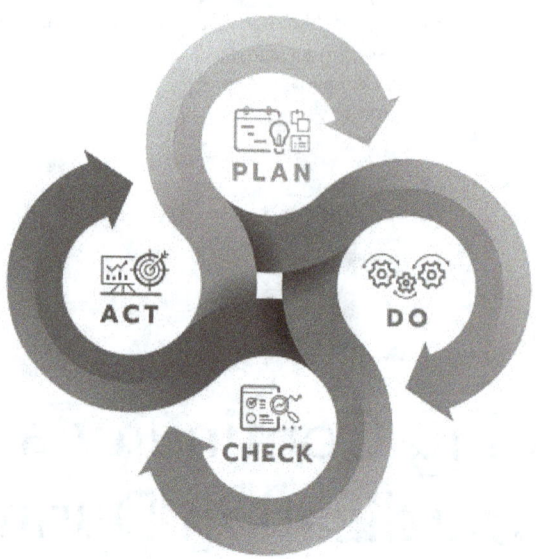

FIGURE 8.1 Plan, Do, Check, Act.

Coupled with the recent organizational trend of healthcare system mergers and acquisitions (778 hospital mergers occurred between 2010 and 2017, resulting in two-thirds of all hospitals being part of a larger system; Gaynor, 2018), mid-level managers were even versed in activities to develop standardization across entities. Yet, the reality of delivering healthcare during a protracted virus remains extremely complex and taxing. Few envisioned this lasting well past two years. Few realized the toll that fatigue, grief, and physical demands would take on healthcare providers, creating a hybrid disaster of a nursing shortage made significantly worse by a pandemic.

Successful organizations were able to use their emergency preparedness plans as a starting point. They were adept at managing rapid-cycle change and were able to roll out new policies and procedures using effective communication, assuring broad acceptance and standardization. They were also able to pivot when something didn't work or new research suggested a better way. In this chapter, we will focus on what made these organizations and leaders better prepared and nimble. We will also discuss the unforeseen challenges and assumptions regarding emergency preparedness, some of which may need re-evaluation for the future.

ORGANIZATIONAL CONTINUITY

Organizational continuity is the ability of a system to continue working during a crisis or disaster. This continuity involves the strategic and tactical ability of an organization to plan for and respond to conditions, situations, and events so that operations are continued at a pre-specified level (DRI International, 2022). It is critical to note that this continuity is impossible without specific pre-planning as introduced in Chapter 7 with the National Incident Management System (NIMS) and the Incident Command System (ICS). Part of this planning is to conduct a hazard vulnerability analysis (EC.4.10, a Joint Commission on Accreditation of Healthcare Organizations [JCAHO] requirement since 2001) to consider all possible disastrous situations and develop strategies to handle the potential issues including physical damage, lack of resources (both personnel and supplies), casualties, interruption of critical services such as water and electricity, and displacement. These could include natural, man-made, and hybrid disasters.

Examples of appropriate pre-planning would include the need for hospitals in the northern US to develop plans for extreme blizzard conditions that could limit the ability for personnel to transit to and from work, possibly interrupt electricity and thus heating abilities and perishable short-stocked items such as fresh food and blood supplies. While there are common disasters and response plans, each facility needs to determine the ones most likely to affect their health system and develop the various contingencies. For example, outside of the western states of Washington, Oregon, and Idaho, most hospitals would not need to have a plan that addressed volcanic eruption.

Public health and hospital system planning for an epidemic was first started following the emergence and then vaccination response to the 1976 novel swine-origin influenza virus. This virus itself did not produce an epidemic, but several critical healthcare needs resulted from both successful and unsuccessful governmental policies attempted at what was viewed as a potential large-scale threat. From this, the first US pandemic plan authored by an interagency group (Centers for Disease Control and Prevention [CDC], National Institutes of Health, Food and Drug Administration, and Department of Defense) was released in 1978 (Iskander et al., 2013). Its plan for pandemic influenza provided recommendations for surveillance, expanded research, established planning and policy mechanisms, and promoted annual influenza immunizations. Several key activities and events led to further refinement of the plan in 1983, followed by significant investments across the globe in collaboration for means to prepare, prevent, and mitigate eventual pandemics. A comprehensive overview of pandemic influenza planning in the United States up to 2008 by Iskander et al. (2013) provides significant historical context to our current public health preparedness plans.

Since 2005, the US Department of Health and Human Services has taken the lead by working with partners in public health, healthcare, and emergency management to improve the nation's pandemic preparedness. The most current pandemic preparedness guidance, plans, and updates are available for download at: https://www.cdc.gov/flu/pandemic-resources/planning-preparedness/national-strategy-planning.html.

Three important assumptions about our previous pandemic planning must be considered, however:

1 The definition of a pandemic has nothing to do with the lethality, possible immunity, or the actual infectious agents. A *pandemic* is defined as "an epidemic occurring worldwide, or over a very wide area, crossing international boundaries and usually affecting a large number of people" (Porta, 2008, p. 179). For hospital systems specifically, preparedness needs to focus on surge capacity and shortage of supplies. Typically, many think of high mortality as being the critical measure, but for maintaining operations during a pandemic crisis, the focus needs to rest on being able to treat the sick who present for care with adequate resources.

2. Most pandemic planning has been dominated by the "influenza" model: "Indeed, 'pandemic' plans at the CDC are explicitly identified as influenza pandemic planning" (Kirlin, 2020, p. 468). Historically, while influenza viruses have produced some of the most significant pandemics, other infectious agents have caused pandemics including human immunodeficiency virus (HIV), Zika, Ebola, Variola major and Variola minor (smallpox), cholera, Yersinia pestis (bubonic plague), and coronaviruses.

Importantly, statistical modeling based on the severity and transmissibility of one pathogen-induced pandemic does not translate to others.

3. Pandemics spread through regions of the world in subsequent waves that are variable with relation to multiple factors such as the exact pathogen, mutations, vaccinations, infection prevention policies, and human behavior (Cacciapaglia et al., 2021). Not having lived through a pandemic of such magnitude and lethality, most healthcare workers were unprepared for this lengthy engagement, nor the resulting variants that emerged.

As we will discuss within this chapter, these factors had large ramifications with the organizational continuity observed over the past two years within healthcare systems, and implications for adapting future emergency preparedness plans. In retrospect, perhaps one of the key words to apply to the pandemic response has been agility. Repeatedly, leaders made decisions, enacted policies and strategies, only to find that something within these measures was not working or that the data revealed something had changed. The media was quick to jump on these trials or resets and label them failures or fumbles. But this mental framework must itself be reset. In an era where all the answers are not known, the trial-and-error approach with decisions made by the brightest minds in the room looking at the big picture is the best approach. True leaders can weather this storm and realize that perhaps 80% of their preplanning, decisions, and approaches to standardization will be correct and result in continuity of care. Research tells us that we make 35,000 decisions each and every day; some of these are bound to be wrong (Sahakian & Labuzetta, 2013). If 20% of the time some aspect is incorrect, then the responsible thing to do is to re-evaluate, reconsider, reset, redeploy. The last thing we should do is to carry on with a policy that is ineffective and dangerous.

In the following section, we will discuss applying change within a crisis, and the frameworks that assist in this change. Central to each is the acceptance that for every change, it is essential that the outcomes are assessed and followed up with either closure of the process with changes firmly ingrained or undertaking a revision and reset to achieve better outcomes.

CHANGE THEORY DURING TIMES OF RAPID MODIFICATION

Effectively managing change is an essential component of healthcare in the age of safety and quality. Several different change models and frameworks have been used in business and healthcare with success. Although change theories are plentiful, including the Deming Plan, Do, Check, Act (Deming Institute, n.d.), here we concentrate on the change theories we found to be most pertinent to the rapid modification required during a pandemic. Table 8.1 outlines the main components of each theory.

MAURER'S RESISTANCE AND CHANGE MODEL

It is almost comical how Maurer categorizes the 3 Levels of Resistance and Change Model (2010) as the basic tenets ring true for most of us in their sheer simplicity. A differentiator to this model is that it focuses on what causes changes to fail. Do the basic premises below even require definition? We have all been there and most likely had to suppress these feelings when changes have come our way. Nonetheless, following are Maurer's 3 Levels of Resistance and Change:

1. **I don't get it**—I don't understand the purpose of the change or how to do it

2. **I don't like it**—Our emotional reaction to the change

3. **I don't like you**—I don't have trust or confidence in you

According to Maurer, the organization's structure can overcome these barriers by:

1. Providing information necessary for change

2. Preparing for and managing roadblocks

3. Remaining confident and informed in the need for change to increase receptiveness

NUDGE THEORY

To "nudge" or prod through indirect encouragement and enablement is the basic premise behind the Nudge Theory developed by American academics Richard Thaler and Cass Sunstein (2008). Nudge Theory is drawn from behavioral economics, political theory, and behavioral sciences to describe the influences in the decisions we make and the design of choices. In short, Nudge Theory is the belief that by shaping the environment, one can influence the likelihood that an individual will choose one option over another. Nudge theory supports that humans have an innate need for heuristic discovery, or the ability to learn something for themselves. Nudge theory supports this need by influencing behavior by allowing the individual to make their own choices, as opposed to directly providing instruction, enforcement, or punishment (Thaler and Sunstein, 2008).

The use of Nudge Theory is based on indirect encouragement and enablement, termed the oxymoronic "libertarian paternalism." Nudge Theory is based on paternalistic recommendations that attempt to steer people in the right direction. The libertarian component is that people are free to resist nudges if they choose to do so. Thus, Nudge Theory attempts to influence, but not require, change (Thaler and Sunstein, 2021).

LEWIN'S CHANGE MODEL THEORY

Lastly, Kurt Lewin's Change Model Theory, most famously known for the precepts to unfreeze, change, and refreeze, suggests that for effective change to occur, three major concepts must be balanced: driving forces, restraining forces, and equilibrium. Driving forces are those that push in a direction for change. They facilitate change and cause a shift in the equilibrium toward a desired direction. Restraining forces counter driving forces and hinder change, pushing in the opposite direction. Equilibrium occurs when driving forces equal restraining forces, and no change occurs (Hussain et al., 2018).

For change to occur, we must find a way to let go of old methods. This is known as unfreezing and will require overcoming individual and group resistance (Hussain et al., 2018). Practical examples of operationalizing unfreezing are to promote effective communication, employee involvement, and training combined with implementing stress management techniques and convincing change reasoning. Unfreezing may be the biggest hurdle, as driving forces must overcome restraining, but once accomplished, it almost seems a relief to proceed with the change. In the final refreezing stage, the change is then established as the new habit, becoming the new norm or tradition.

TABLE 8.1 Change Theory Comparison

Theory	Maurer's Resistance and Change Model	Nudge Theory	Lewin's Change Model Theory
Overview	I don't get it—I don't understand purpose of change or how to do it. I don't like it—Our emotional reaction to the change. I don't like you—I don't have trust or confidence in you.	Subtle, indirect suggestions to nudge people in the direction of the desired change	For effective change to occur, prior learning must be rejected and replaced. Resistance toward the change is overcome during unfreezing. The change is then implemented, and it is solidified into place during refreezing.
Approach	Provide information necessary for change. Prepare for and managing roadblocks. Remain confident and informed in the need for change to increase receptiveness	Define change. Consider employee point of view. Provide evidence to show best options. Present change as a choice. Limit obstacles. Listen to employee feedback. Solidify change with short-term wins to keep up momentum	Unfreeze: Effective communication, conduct needs analysis to determine loopholes, communicate why change needs to occur. Change: Agile and iterative phase to incorporate employee feedback. Refreeze (from transition to acceptance): Identify early adopters and change champions, collect employee feedback regularly

INTEGRATING CHANGE IN THE MIDDLE OF THE PANDEMIC

During the Covid crisis, multiple aspects of daily operations required significant changes to meet the multitude of safety and care needs of providers and patients. Complex decisions were often needed quickly with little or incomplete information. Traditional change management approaches described above by design take a significant amount of time and collaboration. Often, leaders in the pandemic were forced to make an independent decision based on the best knowledge they had at the time and implement a change. The crisis required a shift to a more autocratic leadership style as described by Carson, Vice President of Nursing Practice and Education:

> "Once Covid hit, I had to take more of a directive approach to leadership command and control, to say, 'We're going to do this now; this has to happen.' There's no time for discussion. That's not the best kind of leadership, in my opinion. It burns people out quickly. It's not the right way, particularly in nursing, but sometimes you have to do it. So now I think I'm in a hybrid model depending on what arises. What's the leadership approach I need to take to this to do what's best for the team?"
>
> Carson, Vice President of Nursing Practice and Education

Some changes were more easily undertaken. Specific medical protocols or interventions that were supported by research were quickly adopted. Nancy, a Critical Care Clinical Nurse Specialist, discussed changes with electrolyte protocols and the need for anticoagulation given the hypercoagulable state that was observed in the first few months of the pandemic. Vivian, Critical Care Unit Director, discussed medical care changes based on studies from other countries which observed patient improvement with steroids. Similarly, having experts to assist with supporting the change was crucial:

> "We were so very, very fortunate being here in the metro area and having the [universities] and our epidemiologists so closely connected to our thought leaders and experts at the CDC. We were uniquely positioned and, in some ways, battle tested, because of the involvement with the Ebola outbreak. We had so many experts within our system who were familiar with serious communicable diseases that they also were able to share their expertise. While Covid is not Ebola, those relationships that had been established really, really helped us."
>
> Sharma, Director of Nursing Leadership

The more confounding issue facing our nursing leaders was the need to enact change when the evidence was incomplete and at times conflicting:

> "We all have our ideas about what the workflow should be, what the treatment should be, and when you have very solid literature about how to do something, that's a little bit easier to standardize. But in the absence of solid evidence, everybody just has their own opinion. So, we really had to focus on bringing those opinions together to figure out, even with a lack of evidence, what's the best thing to do. And having to do that without spending weeks and weeks to evaluate. We had to really quickly reach out to others, get examples of what's being done elsewhere, and then figure out how to perform here."
>
> Andrew, Chief Quality Officer in Nursing

While several articles reporting adoption of successful changes during the pandemic have been published, very few in a search of PubMed for 2020 and 2021 discussed employing specific change-management models. Balluck et al. (2020) used the proprietary ADKAR and CLARC Change Models to switch from primary to team nursing during the Covid surge, providing an overview of their change process and communication strategies for the implementation of the change. In another position paper, the Complex Adaptive Systems Model was suggested as a framework to address the unique crisis conditions facing healthcare systems (Choflet et al., 2021). In our opinion, any of the change models or frameworks previously discussed can be used effectively given the adherence to the fundamental leadership processes we've detailed within these chapters. The most important activity is a history of working with the model to enact change throughout times of normalcy so that during times of stress or crisis, the change process is fluid.

THE NEED FOR STANDARDIZATION

During times of crisis, the need for organizational continuity and standardization could not be greater. As discussed in the previous chapter, we recommend an ICS structure for overall direction of the organization. It is important to note here that ICS approaches, including policy and decision-making, should be multilateral in design and structure so they do not become unilateral and hierarchal. There is a danger that hierarchal approaches eliminate engagement of point-of-service stakeholders and experts that can best inform a policy or decision and help assure it is relevant and useful. Designated from the ICS should be uniformly structured practice and logistic teams that can advise and direct care and practice standardization. During a crisis like Covid, where evidence required daily deciphering, policies and procedures were constantly evolving. Effective decisions in a crisis demand local adaptation and customization. There should be evidence of a consistent application of sound policy and evidence-based practices. It would be easy for one unit to make a decision on good evidence and another unit on a different floor of the same hospital to make a non-evidence-based decision for the same patient care procedure. This sets the stage for disequilibrium and issues of safety. Kimberly, Nurse Anesthetist and Nursing Faculty, encountered conflicts with relation to masking requirements in the early days of

Covid between hospitals within the same system. As she described, she encountered a major challenge when implementing changes:

> "Policies made for one hospital didn't translate to others within the system, and it felt like we had to start all over again from scratch every time we went somewhere new."
>
> Kimberly, Nurse Anesthetist and Nursing Faculty

She worked to form an intubation team that was solely responsible for intubating Covid patients all day to minimize donning and duffing and to preserve PPE supply. In the operating room, practice was standardized, and access limited to protect the staff with very strict PPE regulations. Sadly, when she went to the labor and delivery department, they had not implemented any of the organization-wide policies designed to preserve PPE. Nurses and providers were supposed to wear an N-95 mask as well as a level-3 mask on top to preserve the N-95 mask for as long as possible due to the shortage. When she arrived on the labor and delivery unit, level-3 masks were "thrown out everywhere. They were laying around in the hallways and being given, carelessly, to fathers to wear as a normal mask when a surgical mask would have been enough" (Kimberly, Nurse Anesthetist and Nursing Faculty). This set the stage for conflict and ultimately significant time to provide education and direction to the L&D manager and staff to what she had believed were organization-wide rules. This proved to be "one of the most unbelievably frustrating parts." After working to standardize policy adoption with the labor and delivery department, she related that the same thing had to be done in radiology. Because of this lack of organizational continuity, the pace of implementing these protective policies was slowed and resources were not used wisely, which could have compromised patient outcomes and staff safety.

The need was similarly described in a completely different hospital system where this need for standardization was actively being sought:

> "People have an understanding that within that ability to be quick, there must be some level of system-ness and standardization. Otherwise, we won't be able to do those things quickly. If Hospital A is doing something vastly different from Hospital B, we have doctors and nurses and allied health people who are going back and forth between those hospitals because of our staffing issues. If we're doing things differently, everybody's going to be confused. We have the awareness and the understanding that we had to do things in a similar fashion across the entities."
>
> Andrew, Chief Quality Officer in Nursing

FROM PREPARATION TO ADAPTATION

In an article outlining crisis leadership as an opportunity for organizational success, Prewitt and colleagues use a three-phase model (2011). The three phases in a crisis are:

- **Preparation:** A time during which the leader must instill confidence and establish credibility so that their people will be able to phase crisis change in relative safety.

- **Emergency:** Rather than be overcome by the urgency of crisis, the leader takes a step back and makes decisions in line with the organization.

- **Adaptive:** Returns to a sense of stability, and leader will be able to evaluate and address the outcomes and effects of the changes undertaken. Prewitt et al. (2011) note that in this phase there is a delicate balance between maintaining urgency for change while also fostering a sense of safety and security.

In the metropolitan area healthcare systems, the nursing leaders participating in these qualitative interviews described the actions they and their organizations took during the three phases of crisis. Incorporating local historical context, the CDC website, and other articles detailing the response, we have developed a narrative timeline of this response and the leaders' remembrances. We have attempted to highlight specific stories that describe successes and challenges with organizational continuity, rapid-cycle change, and standardization. Embedded within these examples and insights of enacting change during a crisis are key active concepts which by now should be readily articulated with the role of a leader: agility, innovation, decisiveness, communication, and collaboration.

PREPARATION PHASE

All of the healthcare facilities our nurse leaders worked for had emergency preparedness plans containing specific pandemic preparedness, identified surge capacity tenets, and critical resource supply arrangements. These have been accreditation requirements of the JCAHO and the federal government thorough accreditation standards and conditions of participation for the past 30 years.

From the time the first known cases of Covid-19 emerged in China to the first cases in the United States, the timeline of steps taken by the CDC and the World Health Organization (WHO) included the following, constructed from the WHO and CDC historical websites (CDC Museum, 2022; WHO, 2022).

In mid-December 2019, patients in Wuhan, China began to experience symptoms of shortness of breath and fever. By December 31, 2019, WHO had been notified of a large number of cases of pneumonia of unknown etiology in Wuhan. This triggered the activation of the IMS at WHO on January 2, 2020, and a Center Level Response of the CDC for the novel pneumonia. On January 7th, the Chinese government identified and isolated a novel coronavirus as the causative agent, and the CDC established an IMS to guide the response. On January 17th, the CDC began screening passengers on flights from Wuhan to the US, and a team was deployed to Washington state to assist with contact tracing efforts in response to the first reported case of Covid in the US. On January 22nd, human-to-human spread of the virus was confirmed by WHO, and on January 27th, the US Food and Drug Administration announced it was taking critical actions to advance development of novel coronavirus medical countermeasures with interagency partners, including the CDC. By this point, all healthcare facilities had dusted off their emergency response plans and begun leadership discussions concerning the need to activate their ICS. Most began formal meetings and structure the last week of January, when WHO declared the coronavirus outbreak a Public Health Emergency of International Concern and the White House 2019 Novel Coronavirus Task Force was established. Figure 8.2 shows this chronology using a timeline.

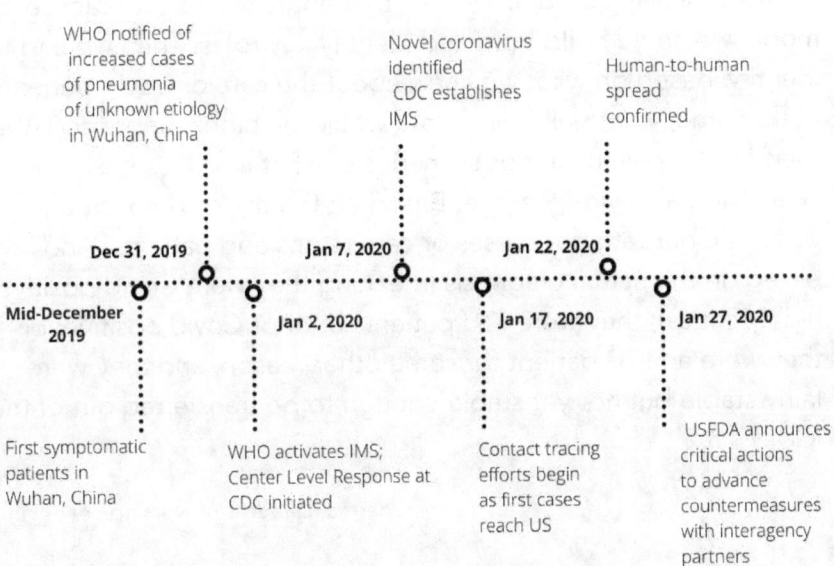

FIGURE 8.2 Steps taken by WHO and the US during the early stages of the Covid-19 pandemic.

In early March 2020, the metropolitan area started to see our first Covid patients. Over the next month, most healthcare facilities moved into the active planning phase for a surge they anticipated would arrive in mid to late spring. Supplies were inventoried, more ordered, and quickly concerns grew concerning the adequacy of existing PPE, ventilators, and certain pharmaceuticals. Care delivery models for the anticipated surge became the highest priority act:

> "My very first assignment was to lead the development of a care delivery model for the surge. Based on data from the experts in infection prevention, we anticipated a surge to happen around the end of April [2020] and what we wanted to do, what the chief nurses wanted to do, was to come up with a way to care for patients in a way that could be standardized across the system. First, we had to pull together a team of representatives from each one of [the] operating units to have representation from each one of those hospitals—critical care nurses because this would be an ICU care delivery model. We had to identify what best practice model we could build from and identify key roles. Then we had to identify, based on what we knew about the care of Covid patients at that time, what skills, what care would be highly prioritized. We then came up with various scenarios of what our ICUs may look like during a Covid-19 surge. Based on the team composition. Based on our ratio for nurses or care teams and patients. And based on the actual diagnosis (meaning they were Covid positive, highly critical; they were ICU patients but not Covid positive; or they were an ICU patient for some other reason, and they were fairly stable but not yet stable enough to be transferred out of the ICU)."
>
> Sharma, Director of Nursing Leadership

Sharma was also engaged with answering the need for additional staff both for the actual surge but also to backfill for nurses exposed to or infected with Covid. Temporary nurse employment contracts were quickly drawn up, and a critical evaluation of existing nursing staff resources was undertaken as described:

> "The chief nurses contracted with nurses who were critical care nurses in pediatrics from the Medical University of South Carolina. We had to identify for those groups of nurses who were going to be brand new to our organization what would be their needs, how we assess their skill sets and their knowledge, how to orient them to our setting. Because of everything that we were seeing and hearing from New York and other places, we knew that getting the staffing right would be a critical component to a successful model. We also looked at what other nurses may be able to support this next group of nurses. We looked at nurses who maybe weren't currently working in ICUs but maybe have some background in emergency nursing or critical care at some point in their career and finding a way to assess what their knowledge, skills, and abilities were. The third layer within this model that we wanted to consider were medical surgical nurses or perhaps nurses who worked in the operating room or an ambulatory care setting who may be able to support the care delivery model either in their current setting or if pulled to an ICU."
>
> Sharma, Director of Nursing Leadership

Nurse leaders described to us the plans put into place for orienting new and travel nurses, cross-training redeployed nurses from one area to another and utilizing team nursing to provide care. The one blessing with the Covid crisis was that there was time to plan. Changes started prior to the first patient's admission in March; however, the surge that most feared did not occur until July.

Successful leadership relies on innovative planning. Seeing the future of possibility but also being able to envision the myriad crises is what enables an organization to navigate the heavy waters of calamity. There is no way to be prepared for every kind of emergency, but to have a plan—a detailed way to move forward in the event of a catastrophe that comes in tandem with the inclusivity, the connections, and the communication that aligns with a vision and with goals—that is effective leadership. It is that partnership and respect that dictates the decision-making process to include all ideas, to creatively pivot in a way that gets everyone to the other side. An effective leader will responsibly admit this is never done alone but is accomplished rather in a continual process that includes other organizations whose goals align with yours and whose shared responsibility is the community of the constituents that you all serve.

EMERGENCY PHASE

On March 14, 2020, Governor Brian P. Kemp signed a public health state of emergency to address novel coronavirus and Covid-19 in Georgia (Office of the Governor, 2020). By this point, 139 people had been diagnosed within Georgia, one person had died, and hospital emergency rooms were starting to see a nervous public concerned that they might be next (Georgia Department of Public Health, 2020). Two weeks later, on Friday, April 3, a statewide shelter in place order went into effect for Georgia, joining a host of other states that were experiencing the same onslaught. Some response plans made according to early (and some would say flawed) guidance were already being followed. Many hospital systems quickly adopted mask policies, requiring staff to wear masks at all times within the facility, but others were slower to do so. This lack of consensus and standardization in initiating mask protocols was met with frustration felt by the nurse leaders we interviewed:

"At some other organizations they were wearing masks already, before we were. Looking back at the beginning, I had to tell staff they couldn't wear masks for regular patient care. That's where we stood: that would make people feel afraid . . . For many things we seem to trail other systems, mask wearing, staff being able to mask the whole time they were in the facility; we were a couple weeks behind in implementing that."

Tanja, Unit Director Labor and Delivery

"[We began with] washing paper gowns and masks and using cloth! And then, 'Put the mask on,' 'Oh no, don't put the mask on,' 'Oh, you know you don't need to wear those masks,' 'It's [going to] be unsafe for you if you put a mask on.' That was the first iteration of mask wearing. Then a month later, 'No, you do need to put the mask on.' So the people who had been chastised during the month that they weren't supposed to be wearing the masks because it was bad for them, are now being told to put the mask on or we are going to chastise you for not putting the mask on!"

Michelle, Innovation and Advancement Coordinator

Timelines for crises do not always turn out as planned. During a crisis, there is often a sense of "hurry up and wait" tension, which cannot be controlled but can be used. In one hospital, the leadership team used this time to pilot an innovative care setting with a smaller number of patients:

"As it turned out, the surge did not come when we expected it, so that gave us the opportunity to pilot the model in certain settings. We were very grateful for the gift of time. The team met consistently from the first week in April through the last week in May (2020) with the understanding that when the surge or predictions changed or if for any reason, we needed to come back together, that we would reconvene to make sure that we had in place what we needed for a safe nursing practice and optimal patient outcomes."

Sharma, Director of Nursing Leadership

Piloting allowed for an extra opportunity to evaluate and adapt the intervention, a notable component of nearly every change model or theory presented earlier in the chapter. Evaluation of the intervention and further refinement is a critical element during any change process. And often what is found is that the change may be adapted into daily routine life following the actual crisis, as observed by Sharma:

"What Covid has taught us in caring for patients, as well as caring for ourselves, is that these models and frameworks that helped strengthen our organization during this crisis will also help in the future as we continue to evaluate the things that we put in place and tweak where we need to tweak. Adapt as needed and if the science changes, really shore up."

Sharma, Director of Nursing Leadership

"It was really just everybody coming together, and it was impressive how quickly, not only those things came through, but how quickly other things came through with people leading them that may not have traditionally led."

Tanja, Unit Director Labor and Delivery

ADAPTIVE PHASE

Two years into the Covid crisis, we understood that this disease would be with us for some time. In Georgia, where these leadership interviews took place, we have had well over 2 million confirmed cases, over 33,000 deaths, and 127,000 hospitalizations related to Covid. We experienced surges in July 2020, January 2021, September 2021, and January 2022. Given the high transmissibility and large number of asymptomatic cases of omicron, the argument can be made that the end of the pandemic is near. By March of 2022, a large portion of the world was infected with the omicron variant, meaning that we have high levels of infection-acquired immunity (Murray, 2022). While the vaccines have proven effective in reducing mortality and hospitalizations, the WHO and CDC are not yet ready to classify Covid as endemic until the number of cases becomes static or stable (Mackintosh & Jani-Friend, 2022).

In terms of crisis response, however, we can look back over the troughs that lie in between the surges as periods of adaption, times when the organization returns to a sense of stability. During this phase, the leader can help the organization re-evaluate, reset, and re-energize. An example of one such opportunity to re-evaluate and reset was with the strict visitation guidelines, put into place during surges, which had detrimental effects on patients and families. Tanja, Unit Director Labor and Delivery, noted:

"Hospital-wide, they're starting to look at the visitor policies again, just because I think we've realized that this is going to be with us for a long time, and we just need some more sustainable practices on how we're going to move forward, because it's not going away."

Tanja, Unit Director Labor and Delivery

The adaptive phase is not necessarily a reversal of urgent policies quickly enacted during the crisis, but rather an appropriate time to re-evaluate and take necessary steps to revise. Revision may take the form of baby steps:

"I think that getting people back on the med-surg floors to be with their elderly family because they are sick—I think about our cancer patients and other similar scenarios; I see them being able to follow our lead and having one visitor . . . before we really go back to fully opening up."

Nancy, Critical Care Clinical Nurse Specialist

This was further articulated by Tanja, Unit Director Labor and Delivery:

"Prior to this, we had a volunteer program where nursing students were coming for 12-hour shifts and providing labor support to people that maybe didn't have somebody with them, or they were planning a natural delivery, or they just could use a little extra support. And so, one of the first things that we want to open back up is getting that program back, because that's a small group of volunteers that we're screening, and they're kind of like our employees, and they're providing a service to us."

Tanja, Unit Director Labor and Delivery

During these periods of adaption, it is critical that leadership allow staff, as well as themselves, time to re-energize and develop resiliency. As we have done throughout this book, taking a deep dive into the choice of a word or phrase, our goal is to better understand the origin and etymology of a word or term that has gone viral, but perhaps is not fully appreciated: resilience.

Resilience has Latin roots and originally was used in the 1600s with the now obsolete definition of "the action or an act of rebounding or springing back; rebound, recoil." We now use this term to describe the human capacity to be "able to recover quickly or easily from, or resist being affected by a misfortune, shock, illness, etc." (Oxford English Dictionary, 2021). Carson, one of our more senior leaders, is devoting his energies to helping his organization assure that in these periods of adaption, resilience is fostered:

> "Resilience needs to rest on the shoulders of health systems and leaders. Currently, resilience rests on the shoulders of individual nurses, and we need to move away from that system. It's important as leaders for us to create safe spaces for our teams to practice resilience and self-care in the work setting. And if we don't do that as leaders, then we'll never see the resilience that we expect of our nurses."
>
> — Carson, Vice President of Nursing Practice and Education

Allowing for resilience must be a central component of the adaptive phase of emergency response. Fostering resilience must become engrained within our emergency response planning in order to allow our most critical team members to react to stress in a healthy way through which goals are achieved at a minimal psychological and physical cost (Epstein & Krasner, 2013). Going forward, this could translate into actual written actions within the emergency response plan devoted to the care of the physical and mental health of nurses and other healthcare professionals. Placing a priority on addressing the emotional toll that accompanies acting in a climate of pressure, fear, and uncertainty. Carson concluded by focusing on the need to foster resilience as a priority as healthcare facilities transition from a disaster caused by a pathogen to a crisis of personnel:

"We're doing a lot of retention programs for our nurses. We've done some system-wide resilience programs to encourage resilience building. I meet with nurse leaders to try to work with them to see if there are ways that they can provide more space and time for self-care and resilience for their nurses. We do close follow-up with our nurses that we have concern about or who express wanting to leave. And we have systems in place so that a nurse feeling burnout working on ICU, rather than leaving, [we] might see if we can get them on another unit, such as an emergency setting. Maybe they want to try an OB Labor and Delivery Unit. We have systems developed within the hospital to try to move people around to get them what they need so they can be their best selves. We're having to certainly amplify a lot of that work right now."

Carson, Vice President of Nursing Practice and Education

ADAPTABILITY AND HIGH RELIABILITY ORGANIZATIONS

High reliability organizations (HROs) are noted for their ability to avoid catastrophes in the face of high levels of risk and organizational complexity. These organizations by necessity are required to be focused on risk because of their exceptionally high capacity for positive and negative human impact. Organizations such as nuclear power plants, aircraft carriers, air traffic control systems, petroleum plants, city water systems, etc. are examples of such systems. High reliability organizations are of special interest because of their amazing capacity to succeed in their service with regularity and with few or no failing systems. Examination of the systems yielded five critical factors that directly relate to their success in avoiding the potential for disaster (Oster & Braaten, 2021; Weick & Sutcliff, 2001):

1. Preoccupation with failure
2. Reluctance to simplify
3. Sensitivity to operations
4. Commitment to resilience
5. Deference to expertise

PRINCIPLE 1: PREOCCUPATION WITH FAILURE

Many organizations either ignore or look past small process challenges or limitations. An HRO cannot. These systems do not overlook any potential for failure no matter how small it might be or inconsequential a deviation might result and immediate address any level of human or technical process failures. Even if the issue is preliminary or not yet potentially dangerous, the HRO reviews it closely, giving the impression that they are preoccupied with failures. This requires the HRO train and develop all workers in every level of the system to see as their personal obligation any possibility or indication that something needs to be addressed. All staff, regardless of their role, are expected to report any unusual or suspected circumstances in a manner that widely distributes information and assures organizational transparency at every level.

PRINCIPLE 2: RELUCTANCE TO SIMPLIFY

Because HROs are definitively complex, they embrace the complexity and accept all the implications embedded in it. Leaders in the systems expect employees to have some element of risk and to challenge the organization's attention and integrity. No problem is too small to be addressed, explained away, or analyzed. Root cause analysis is a fundamental part of problem identification and solution seeking as the HRO attempts to maintain systems homeostasis. Leaders in these environments continually challenge past practices, policies, assumptions, and belief systems.

These leaders continuously respond to data and build evidence grounded approaches, benchmarks, and performance metrics. Indeed, a significant leadership skill set is the capacity to constantly seek information that challenges the status quo and provide opportunity for problem identification, innovation, and problem solving (Weick & Sutcliff, 2001).

PRINCIPAL 3: SENSITIVITY TO OPERATIONS

Leaders in these models recognize the importance of each element of the system and every person within the organization. Hierarchies are diminished and collateral communication networks that engage all players in the HRO system are the common organizational structure. These leaders understand that those who spend their work lives on the front lines of the organization are likely the first line of information and access to the potential for problems and for opportunities for solutions and necessary changes. These leaders not only respect all members of the work team, they actively seek engagement, information, and full participation in problem solving from all stakeholders. The practice of regular visits to all work assignments by leaders is common in HROs and is considered a high reliability practice (Weick & Sutcliff, 2001).

PRINCIPLE 4: COMMITMENT TO RESILIENCE

Predictive and adaptive characteristics are idealized in HROs. The capacity of leaders and staff includes not only anticipating the potential for trouble but expecting it as a part of the normal operations of HROs. These organizations must be able to identify the potential for problems early and eagerly seek innovative solutions that can respond easily to change. This means leaders must create a dynamic environment that responds quickly to challenge and change well in front of emergencies in an ongoing effort to maintain the stability and integrity of the system. In order to foster this resilience, HROs depend broadly on cross referenced multidisciplinary teams in an attempt to remove any barriers to collaboration and communication. Flexibility and readiness to change and adapt to shifting conditions, resources, or circumstances is a critical element of personal and organizational success. Resilient team members remain so because they are explicitly trained on anticipating and managing unexpected events (Weick & Sutcliff, 2001).

PRINCIPLE 5: DEFERENCE TO EXPERTISE

In HROs, expertise is highly valued. Organizational charts include the value role of expertise as one of the sources of authority and legitimacy in the organization structure. Competency in content expertise that demonstrates deep, subject knowledge and applications are considered of exceptionally high value. Such competencies are then used as an operational norm for maintaining stability in the organization and for assessment and urgent response to situational issues and concerns. Specialty knowledge is clearly enumerated in the functional expectations, and utilization of a particular knowledge base and skill set is a feature of the work structure and relationships in HROs. In addition, continuing education, development, and refinement of knowledge and skills is considered a part of the work role and incorporated into the activities of workers. Here again, team relationships and knowledge crossover and integration are critical to the viability and success of HROs since solutions are often found at the intersection between various levels of expertise, and innovative solutions only emerge from expert interactions (Weick & Sutcliff, 2001).

NURSES NEED ORGANIZATIONAL STABILITY

In part, people come and go from organizations based on their personal fit within that culture and how adaptive organizations can be to pressing demands—whether caused by a natural crisis in the form of Covid-19 to now a hybrid crisis of the nursing shortage as a result of the pandemic. Sadly for the nursing profession, this revolving door is spinning a little too quickly. Various reported statistics exist, from a projection of 22% of bedside professional nurses leaving the bedside in 2022 (Berlin et al., 2021), to an alarming finding that the median length of tenure for an RN in a clinical position is 2.78 years (Thayer et al., 2022) compared to an average of 4.4 years for other hourly compensated, comparable positions. The staggering nursing shortage of 1.1 million nurses (American Nurses Association, n.d.), fosters this turnover, allowing nurses to hop from institution to the next for lack of fit, until they find a better match. This practice is costly for the employers because the investment in training and orientation may not be recouped, and it prevents the unit or department from cohesively working on issues to better the environment. Critical to change success in a crisis (or during routine times) is the presence of a stable, cohesive team and a culture that can adapt through agile leadership, valuing contributions, communication, and systematic evaluation.

Nursing professionals have an elevated level of accountability for creating an environment of safety, healing, and hope. This accountability indicates a need for shared decisions and actions in responding to crisis and undertaking change. This ownership implies that the professional nursing staff can count on leaders engaging staff in collateral and collegial problem solving, solution seeking, idea generating, shared decision-making, and responsive action. The professional staff should be seen by leadership as partners in the process of responding to crisis who can advance new ways of thinking and acting as well as create innovative approaches to patient care in the presence of limitations, challenges, and uncertainty. Leaders who do not both recognize and live inside of this partnership with the professional nursing staff become another causative element contributing to fear, anxiety, isolation, disenfranchisement, and ultimately, hopelessness and burnout. Communication means not only sharing information transparently, it also means advancing personal investment and engagement with professional nursing partners essential to the resolution of the crisis.

Leaders must be authentic and transparent in their relationship with those they lead. Leaders must know themselves as people and as leaders. Staff cannot legitimately look at leaders as though they have superpowers and are able to do things beyond ordinary understanding. When any individuals are placed on a platform of exceptionalism, given sufficient time, they will either fall off or be knocked off. Idealizing leaders beyond human norms ultimately creates certain failure or downfall.

It is the obligation of the leader to first recognize their own humanity. This includes a level of personal clarity about emotional strengths and challenges, what is known and not known, and how this individual engages others' strengths to supplement their own in a way that facilitates a collective community of wisdom and action. This confluence of personal characteristics becomes a powerful tool, evidencing the good leader is essentially an effective relationship builder, always aware of the strengths and gifts of others as well as their vulnerabilities and needs. The effective leader embraces vulnerability and makes it a tool for relationship building and leadership effectiveness. In so doing, leaders reflect on the staff the value of that vulnerability in a way that accelerates leaders' own capacity to include, engage, and embrace the team in problem solving, solution seeking, and supporting the relationships and efforts of the team.

We saw this level of personal insight, self-resilience, and ability to self-correct with Carson, our VP of Nursing Practice and Education. Carson had worked in Africa with patients dying of Ebola in a previous position. He shared with us his ability to recognize his own emotional struggles that surfaced with Covid and how this sometimes interfered with his ability to stay focused and communicate effectively. But he was able to self-correct and ultimately lead with humility, strength, and confidence. He acknowledged:

"One of my big weaknesses is that I still have some PTSD from when I treated Ebola patients. I lost count of the deaths that we saw. Every day, just people dying right and left or you would walk into work and be surrounded by dead bodies. Horrible, horrible. And so, as Covid started to ramp up, my PTSD kicked in and I went into emergency mode as I have to do this now, and this now, and this now. And that became a little too much, I think, for myself, some of my colleagues, because I was a little scatterbrained about it. So that was certainly a weakness. Other weaknesses were learning the communication structures, assuming that if we've made this decision, we're going to communicate it with these groups, assuming that was enough. And then we'd roll something out, think it is rolled out, and then a week later it is still not happening because I did not help guide the communication, the way it needed to go. Very rarely are we right most of the time, especially in a time of a crisis where no one knows what is going on. That was a big lesson that I'm still trying to learn is vulnerability—how to be with that [vulnerability] and how to really listen to my teams."

Carson, Vice President of Nursing Practice and Education

KEY TAKEAWAYS

Every organization has a specific culture, defined as the "deeper level of basic assumption and beliefs that are shared by the members of an organization that operate unconsciously and define in a basic taken-for-granted fashion an organization's view of itself and its environment" (Schein, 1992). Central to a culture is having standards or norms. Most older nurses remember going to a new institution and learning the "[Insert Institution Name Here] Way." Whether it was how a dressing was changed, an IV taped securely, or daily weights done, there was always a slightly different way to do things here versus there. Every healthcare entity had established their own policies and procedures for actions, both written and unwritten. As clinical professional nurses who delivered bedside care from the 1970s to 2000s, we understand the root problem of this divergence was that practice standards did not exist then. But by 2014, 55% of all nursing practices were based on research findings, and by last year, the ANA had predicted that 90% of all nursing practice would be based in research (Chrisman et al., 2014). A critical learning is that, when possible, change must be based on the best evidence, communicated effectively, standardized across an institution, and then critically evaluated with swift modifications, without apology, as necessary.

In the next chapter, we will take a deeper dive into the role of the leader in caring for their team during a crisis as well as during times of normalcy. We'll evaluate how caring, protectionism, and fostering of resiliency are demonstrated and realized along with determining the correct amounts. Can there be too much?

REFLECTIVE EXERCISES

8.1 → CORRECTING COURSE

Reflect on a project that was not going according to plan, or for which unforeseen complications developed. In modifying the plan, you fear your team will question your capability and decision-making about the original change and will not trust your proposed modifications. Discuss the following aspects:

- Identify the original change.

- What were the complications?

- How did you decide to make corrections?

- What were your strategies in deploying the correction that were effective and built trust?

- What did you learn from this and how will you proceed in a future situation like this?

_____

_____

_____

_____

_____

_____

_____

_____

8.2 → EXPLORING THE DISCOMFORT OF CHANGE

We have a little exercise that involves some physical movement: Cross your arms. Now that you are comfortable, cross your arms the other way. Why was the second attempt more uncomfortable, even though it's basically the same action?

So now for your reflective exercise, consider a specific change being made within your organization. Examine how tricky it is to cross your arms in different positions and equally how tricky it is to cope with change.

- Identify a change being made in your organization.
- How do you feel about it?
- What are you being asked to change?

8.3 → AREA OF IMPROVEMENT

Using the STARR technique, describe a specific change that needed to occur during the pandemic. Then identify the tasks involved, what actions you took, the result of those actions, and what you might do differently in the future.

Situation Describe the challenging situation.	
Task Describe the task at hand or target desired.	
Action Describe the actions taken and possibly the alternatives available.	
Result Describe the outcome of your actions, including the ability to meet your objective.	
Reflection What did you learn? What would you do differently, the same, or better next time being posed with a similar situation?	

8.4 → HIGH RELIABILITY ORGANIZATION

Is your organization an HRO? Reflect on how your organization is committed to the five principles discussed in the text. How do you personally support the HRO, and what as a leader can you do better?

Principles	How Your Organization Demonstrates Commitment	How Do You Personally Support?	What Areas Can Be Improved?
Preoccupation with failure			
Reluctance to simplify			
Sensitivity to operations			
Commitment to resilience			
Deference to expertise			

REFERENCES

American Nurses Association. (n.d.). *Nurses in the workforce.* https://www.nursingworld.org/practice-policy/workforce/

Balluck, J., Asturi, E., & Brockman, V. (2020). Use of the ADKAR® and CLARC® change models to navigate staffing model changes during the COVID-19 pandemic. *Nurse Leader, 18*(6), 539–546. https://doi.org/10.1016/j.mnl.2020.08.006

Berlin, G., Lapointe, M., Murphy, M., & Viscardi, M. (2021, May 11). Nursing in 2021: Retaining the healthcare workforce when we need it most. *McKinsey & Company.* https://www.mckinsey.com/industries/healthcare-systems-and-services/our-insights/nursing-in-2021-retaining-the-healthcare-workforce-when-we-need-it-most

Cacciapaglia, G., Cot, C., & Sannino, F. (2021). Multiwave pandemic dynamics explained: How to tame the next wave of infectious diseases. *Scientific Reports, 11*, 6638. https://doi.org/10.1038/s41598-021-85875-2

CDC Museum. (2022). *COVID-19 timeline.* https://www.cdc.gov/museum/timeline/covid19.html

Choflet, A., Packard, T., & Stashower, K. (2021). Rethinking organizational change in the COVID-19 era. *Journal of Hospital Management and Health Policy, 5.* https://doi.org/10.21037/jhmhp-21-11

Chrisman, J., Jordan, R., Davis, C., & Williams, W. (2014). Exploring evidence-based practice research. *Nursing Made Incredibly Easy!, 12*(4), 8–12. doi: 10.1097/01.NME.0000450295.93626.e7

Demings Institute. (n.d.). *PDSA cycle.* https://deming.org/explore/pdsa/

DRI International. (2022). *International glossary for resilience.* https://drii.org/resources/glossary

Epstein, R. M., & Krasner, M. S. (2013). Physician resilience: What it means, why it matters, and how to promote it. *Academic Medicine, 88*(3), 301–303. https://doi.org/10.1097/acm.0b013e318280cff0

Gaynor, M. (2018). *Examining the impact of health care consolidation.* Committee on Energy and Commerce Oversight and Investigations Subcommittee. https://docs.house.gov/meetings/IF/IF02/20180214/106855/HHRG-115-IF02-Wstate-GaynorM-20180214.pdf

Georgia Department of Public Health. (2020). *Covid-19 status report.* https://dph.georgia.gov/covid-19-status-report

Hussain, S., Akram, T., Haider, M., Hussain, S., & Ali, M. (2018). Kurt Lewin's change model: A critical review of the role of leadership and employee involvement in organizational change. *Journal of Innovation and Knowledge, 3*(3), 123–127. https://doi.org/10.1016/j.jik.2016.07.002

Iskander, J., Strikas, R. A., Gensheimer, K. F., Cox, N. J., & Redd, S. C. (2013). Pandemic influenza planning, United States, 1978–2008. *Emerging Infectious Diseases, 19*(6), 879–885. https://doi.org/10.3201/eid1906.121478

Kirlin, J. (2020). COVID-19 upends pandemic plan. *The American Review of Public Administration, 50*(6–7), 467–479. https://doi.org/10.1177/0275074020941668

Mackintosh, E., & Jani-Friend, I. (2022, January 19). Covid pandemic "nowhere near over," WHO says. *CNN.com*. https://www.cnn.com/2022/01/19/world/coronavirus-newsletter-intl-01-19-22/index.html

Maurer, R. (2010). *Beyond the wall of resistance: Why 70% of all changes fail and what you can do about it* (Revised ed.). Bard Press.

Murray, C. J. L. (2022). COVID-19 will continue but the end of the pandemic is near. *Lancet, 399*(10323), 417–419. https//doi.org/10.1016/S0140-6736(22)00100-3

Office of the Governor, Governor Brian P. Kemp. (2020, March 16). *Kemp declares public health state of emergency*. https://gov.georgia.gov/press-releases/2020-03-16/kemp-declares-public-health-state-emergency

Oster, C., & Braaten, J. (2021). *High reliability organizations*. Sigma Theta Tau International.

Oxford English Dictionary. (2021). *Resilience*. In Oxford English Dictionary online. https://www-oed-com

Porta, M. (Editor). (2008). *A dictionary of epidemiology* (5th ed.). Oxford University Press.

Prewitt, J. E., Weil, R. S., & McClure, A. Q. (2011). Crisis leadership – An organizational opportunity. *Australian Journal of Business and Management Research, 1*(6), 60–74.

Sahakian, B. J., & Labuzetta, J. N. (2013). *Bad moves: How decision making goes wrong, and the ethics of smart drugs*. Oxford University Press.

Schein, E. (1992). *Organizational culture and leadership* (2nd ed.). Jossey-Bass Publishers.

Thaler, R. H., & Sunstein, C. R. (2008). *Nudge: Improving decisions about health, wealth, and happiness*. Penguin Books.

Thaler, R. H., & Sunstein, C. R. (2021). *Nudge: The final edition*. Penguin Books.

Thayer, J., Zillmer, J., Sanberg, N., Miller, A. R., Nagel, P., & MacGibbon, A. (2022). "The new nurse" is the new normal. *Epic Research*. https://epicresearch.org/articles/the-new-nurse-is-the-new-normal

Weick, K. E., & Sutcliffe, K. M. (2001). *Managing the unexpected: Assuring high performance in an age of complexity*. Jossey-Bass.

World Health Organization. (2022). *Timeline: WHO's COVID-19 response.* https://www.who.int/emergencies/diseases/novel-coronavirus-2019/interactive-timeline#event-2

"I can be changed by what happens to me. But I refuse to be reduced by it."
—**Maya Angelou, poet**

9

Coping, Resilience, and Posttraumatic Growth

Researchers originally began warning of the long-lasting emotional trauma from the Covid-19 crisis in the first few months of it reaching the shores of the United States, recognizing the combined unique features of a global pandemic causing fear, isolation, economic instability, and the extremes of illness and loss of life (Higgins, 2020). Within nursing, surveys completed during the first year of the pandemic by the International Council of Nurses (ICN, 2021a) reported that the nursing workforce had experienced extreme trauma.

In January 2021, over 2,200 nurses had succumbed to Covid-19, and 80% of nurses worldwide reported mental distress. Within the US, the American Nurses Association

> **WE ASKED NURSE LEADERS**
>
> → Who supported you in the organization?
>
> → What are you/your unit/ your hospital doing to support your staff holistically during the Covid-19 crisis?
>
> → How did you feel about being overwhelmed?
>
> → When you were flying by the seat of your pants, can you identify one thing you did to deal with the crisis?

reported that 51% of nurses felt "overwhelmed," while other reports suggested 93% of healthcare workers were experiencing stress, 76% reported exhaustion and burnout, as alarmingly, nurse-to-patient ratios had increased threefold (ICN, 2021a). Just 10 months later, the ICN released a follow-up report that an estimated 115,000 healthcare workers worldwide had died as a direct result of the Covid pandemic (ICN, 2021b).

These figures are extremely troublesome when considering, pre-pandemic, there was a gap in the nursing workforce of six million. Now, with the mass exodus of the nurses we touched on at the end of Chapter 8, we are facing a 13 million nurse deficit by 2030 (ICN, 2021b). Recently, Nurse.org released a report of the state of nursing (2022), drawing on interviews with 1,500 nurses across the country. Importantly, these surveys were undertaken with RNs, nurse practitioners, and APRNS, and revealed a professional discipline struggling. In one year, the number of nurses reporting they felt burned out had risen to 87%, with 84% reporting they felt frustrated with administration, were underpaid, and that their mental health was suffering. Sadly, 77% reported feeling unsupported at work, 61% felt unappreciated, and 58% felt unsafe at work. It is no wonder then that only 12% of the nurses surveyed reported feeling satisfied with their current work situation (Nurse.org, 2022).

In this chapter, looking from the perspective of innovation, we will strive to understand the key factors of crisis, trauma, coping, and posttraumatic growth (PTG) theory and address specific tactics leaders can employ to foster resilience and PTG on a personal level as well as with their teams.

TRAUMA AND ITS OUTCOMES

The American Psychological Association (APA) defines trauma as "an emotional response to a terrible event like an accident, rape or natural disaster" (APA, 2022b, para. 1). Trauma affects everyone and every organization differently, depending on numerous contextual factors, including the meaning of the trauma, type of trauma experienced, individual and organizational characteristics, and sociocultural factors, among others. Typically, the initial symptoms are shock and denial that the event happened, and/or that it affected the person. Later, the person may experience negative alterations in thinking and mood, flashbacks and other intrusive experiences, hyperarousal, and avoidance (APA, 2013).

If these symptoms persist and cause difficulty, this response is considered posttraumatic stress disorder (PTSD). Those with PTSD may feel stressed or frightened even when not in danger. These distressing symptoms often feel involuntary, intrusive, and deeply uncomfortable. While experiencing trauma is a common occurrence, PTSD is rare. It is more common for individuals to exhibit brief symptoms or even resilient responses to experiencing trauma. This speaks to our remarkable potential for resiliency and growth, and previous research has demonstrated that even the most traumatic experiences among individuals and organizations can lead to positive reactions.

RESILIENCY

Resiliency has several conceptualizations but is generally described as the ability to bounce back from difficulty, or to adapt in such a way that people can adjust to difficulties they face (Luthar et al., 2000; Rutter, 1985). While early researchers described resilience as being a trait, as in "either you have it or you don't," the vast proliferation in recent work on resiliency's influencing role in mental health promotion and overall well-being points to the ability to influence and even foster resiliency, thus classifying resiliency as a skill. This can also be conceptualized as a bounce forward, describing highly resilient individuals as less likely to experience future struggles as they learn to navigate difficulty and adapt to future stressors (Haas, 2015). Leys and colleagues argue that since resilience can be degraded and fostered, it is crucial to both "better understand the underlying processes of resilience and to put in place interventions that target these processes" (2020, p. 5). Specific to the Covid pandemic response, resiliency has been identified as a promising buffer in decreasing negative psychological impact of the pandemic, with diminished depression, anxiety, and burnout among healthcare workers (Finstad et al., 2021).

POSTTRAUMATIC GROWTH

Nurse leaders navigating through this crisis must prioritize a sense of resiliency for themselves and their teams in the aftermath of this devastating period (Cunningham & Pfeiffer, 2022). This may seem an insurmountable challenge while also enduring the acute-now-chronic toll of this pandemic, which has upended so many of our very core assumptions about what we thought to be true and reliable about ourselves, our world, and our healthcare systems/work environments. It may feel impossible to make sense of the aftermath of this crisis and find what good could possibly come from the trauma we have endured. A theoretical framework developed by Tedeschi and Calhoun (1995), PTG describes the positive psychological and transformative changes that arise from the very disruptions that upend our understanding of our anticipated life course. The construct of PTG suggests that it is the upending—and its subsequent struggle, reassessment, and rebuilding that arises from such disorientation—which fosters growth.

PTG has been recognized to occur in five domains (Tedeschi & Calhoun, 1995). Persons experiencing a trauma or crisis can develop:

1. Improved relationships with others
2. A greater sense of personal strength
3. Openness to new possibilities
4. A stronger sense of spirituality or existential growth
5. A greater appreciation of life

Research using a self-report instrument called the Posttraumatic Growth Inventory has found strong evidence for PTG across many cultures and populations, including healthcare workers facing occupationally driven traumatic experiences (Tedeschi et al., 2018). Table 9.1 provides the context and affirmations for each domain.

TABLE 9.1 Five Domains of Posttraumatic Growth

Domain	Context	Affirmation
Relating to Others	Positive changes in relationships	"I appreciate"
New Possibilities	New paths, interests, and opportunity	"I dream"
Personal Strength	Self-reliance, confidence, and a sense of perseverance	"I am able to"
Spiritual/Existential Change	Deeper connections and reflections with spiritual and existential matters	"I accept"
Appreciation for Life	Gratitude for things life has to offer	"I cherish" or "I notice"

Tedeschi et al., 2018

PTG differs from resilience in that resiliency is a common ability to endure and move forward in response to crisis, but PTG involves growth beyond pre-trauma levels of coping (Tedeschi et al., 2018). Highly resilient people may not face such a challenge that forces reimagining of perspectives and beliefs that shape our approach to living. Research differs on the relationship between resilience and PTG, but the strategies to support each overlap considerably. Importantly, distress, PTSD, and other psychological difficulties can coexist alongside resilience and PTG (Schubert et al., 2016).

COPING

Coping is the ability to manage internal and external stressors. The American Psychological Association defines it as "the use of cognitive and behavioral strategies to manage the demands of a situation when these are appraised as taxing or exceeding one's resources or to reduce the negative emotions and conflict caused by stress" (APA, 2022a, para. 1). There are multiple theories, strategies, and models of coping, with tomes written about them that are beyond the spectrum of this chapter. In general, we want to emphasize that coping plays a major role in the development of PTG or resiliency (Prati & Pietrantoni, 2009). Coping can be adaptive, thereby improving functioning and contribute to resilience and/or PTG, or maladaptive, which is generally unhelpful in the long term. There are internal and external factors that influence coping. These are outlined in Table 9.2.

TABLE 9.2 Internal and External Coping Factors

Internal Coping Factors	External Coping Factors
Self-efficacy	Social support
Emotional regulation	Family and friends
Confidence	Camaraderie
Sense of belonging	Professional support from therapists, clergy, or medical practitioners
Interpersonal skills	
Self-acceptance	
Help-seeking and receiving behaviors	

Importantly, coping and resulting resilience or PTG are related but are different constructs. Resilience refers to the ability to recover from a stressful event (Luthar et al., 2000; Rutter, 1985); PTG involves growth beyond pre-trauma levels of coping; and coping itself refers to active employment of cognitive and behavioral strategies to manage the stressful event (Folkman & Moskowitz, 2004).

COPING STRATEGIES AND IMPLICATIONS FOR POSITIVE CHANGE

→ Adaptive coping is derived from a variety of personal and environmental factors.

→ Key strategies that influence development of resilience and PTG are positive appraisal and social support.

→ Leaders can support themselves and their teams by deliberately fostering a supportive work environment.

→ Organizations should prioritize interventions to support active coping.

DELIBERATE REFLECTION

Whether an unexpected tornado has destroyed everything in its path, or a healthcare system infrastructure has been damaged, crises result in challenges to our ability to understand what has happened and where to rebuild. Recall that often, in the aftermath of a traumatic experience, recollection can feel intrusive and unresolved and is a stressful (though normal) response. On the other hand, deliberate, reflective practice on the domains of PTG can be viewed as an ongoing process improvement plan to understand the progression of PTG among individuals and in organizational culture (Cunningham & Pfeiffer, 2022).

It is this shift in the cognitive struggle with trauma that plays a key role in PTG development. Deliberate reflection, also referred to as deliberate rumination, occurs when individuals, organizations, systems, and communities engage in conscious efforts to rebuild, integrating the trauma into the new story. The positive association between this type of action-oriented, thoughtful reflection and PTG is well documented (Hill & Watkins, 2017; Hirooka et al., 2017; Stockton et al., 2011).

The idea that growth comes out of adversity is not new; this is a centuries-old idea present in cultures worldwide: the rebirth of the phoenix, warrior's journey, and the philosophical idea of strength over pain coined by Friedrich Nietzsche's famous quote: "Was mich nicht umbringt macht mich stärker" ("That which does not kill me makes me stronger"). Tedeschi et al. (2018) explain that this type of transcendent growth is attributed to a variety of processes, and the phenomenon of PTG is related to and derived from many other theoretical models relevant for clinical application, including those on coping, appraisal, and change in response to crises (Janoff-Bulman, 1989; Lazarus & Folkman, 1984; Schaefer & Moos, 1992; Zoellner & Maercker, 2006). This helps explain how intentionally reconstructing thinking about the trauma event can form a solid contextual foundation of growth in the aftermath.

Table 9.3 provides the outcome domains of PTG and guiding questions for deliberate reflection to contemplate possible evolution in both the leader and the organization.

TABLE 9.3 Reflections on PTG Domains Following the Pandemic

Domain	Individual	Organizational
Relating to Others	Who do you count on in difficult times? Which relationships have become stronger and more connected? Who do you look to for perspective around surviving this event?	What have other organizations done when coming through similar difficulty? Are we prioritizing honest and open team dialogue?
New Possibilities	What new interests and ideas have you developed because of the pandemic? What can you learn from this experience?	What lessons from this crisis have or will spark innovation? In what ways are we improving workflows and where have we been stuck in processes that no longer serve our mission? Are we holding space for creativity and new ideas?

Personal Strength	Where do you notice your confidence? What new challenges are you managing? From where and whom do you draw strength?	What are we doing well? Where can we leverage across teams to support and foster existing strengths? Who are our role models?
Spiritual/ Existential Change	How do you perceive your life's plan? How have your spiritual, religious, or existential perspectives shifted? Where and with whom do you find harmony?	What are our true values? Do they align with our vision, mission, community, and teamwork approach?
Appreciation for Life	Have your priorities changed about what is most important in your life and work? Do you have greater appreciation for the value of your life or notice aspects you no longer take for granted?	How do we demonstrate appreciation for the team/ employees? Is there a plan in place for fostering a culture of well-being?

(Adapted from Cunningham & Pfeiffer, 2022; Maitlis, 2020; Olson et al., 2020; Tedeschi et al., 2018)

These PTG Domains are also underscored in the adaptability concepts presented in Chapters 3 and 4, which can facilitate adaptive coping via nurturing leadership by fostering conditions for PTG. Figure 9.1 depicts a very simplified hypothesis of the role of coping and perceived support in fostering PTG and resilience adapted from these theoretical concepts, incorporating Tedeschi et al.'s (2018) Revised Model of Posttraumatic Growth. What follows is a series of recommendations aimed at facilitating such factors for ourselves as leaders, and for our healthcare teams.

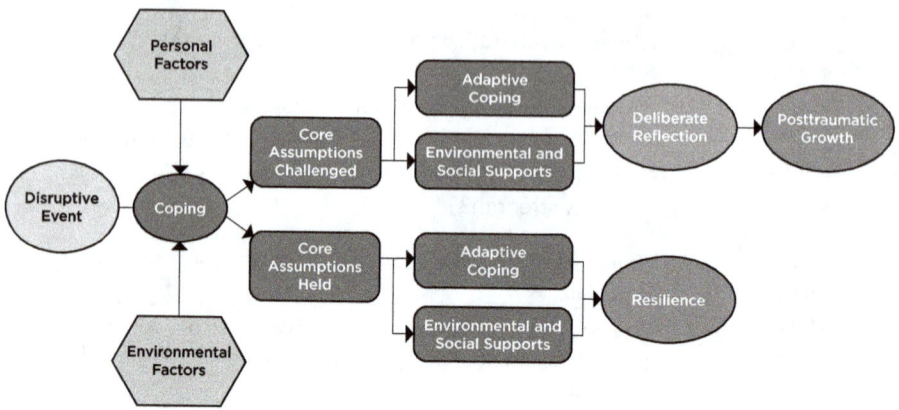

FIGURE 9.1 A perspective on the role of coping in fostering positive outcomes to trauma.

FOSTERING ADAPTIVE COPING TO ENHANCE POSITIVE CHANGE

Notably, it is not the trauma event itself that solely determines outcomes for an individual, team, or organization, but rather the struggle we go through with interpreting and ascribing meaning to our most terrible experiences that shapes PTG. The seismic shift in pandemic-driven leadership has forced a new path in the wake of our collective trauma experience. There is simply no going back to the old way of doing things. In a PTG approach, traumatic stress is not solely potentially devastating; it is also a great catalyst for transformative individual and organizational change. The active improvement process of facilitating adaptive coping to cultivate deliberate reflection can be challenging but important work to shape PTG and use the disruption to propel healing and evolution for leaders and their teams, colleagues, or loved ones (Olson et al., 2020; Tedeschi et al., 2018). These clinicians may have encountered various challenges, such as not having enough personal protective equipment, being assigned to practice in areas outside their expertise, dealing with a lack of known therapeutics, making difficult decisions about rationing or prioritizing care, and facing disruptions affecting many aspects of healthcare and daily life. This acute stress among healthcare professionals is superimposed on preexisting high levels of occupationally related psychological and occupational stress.

FOSTERING PTG IN LEADERS

However horrific the experiences faced as leaders and healthcare workers, there lies the ability to adapt and grow stronger, and use this growth to help healthcare teams do the same. Leaders must foster these concepts within themselves in order to enculturate growth among teams. No one was immune to the trauma induced by Covid, and while many leaders have put on a brave face and have perhaps used avoidance coping as a means to power through, we must support these positive traits within ourselves.

> **QUALITIES OF COPING CHECKLIST**
> Ask yourself! Is it:
>
> - ❏ Helpful
> - ❏ Optimistic
> - ❏ Flexible
> - ❏ Action oriented
> - ❏ Focused on a shared goal
> - ❏ Socially inclusive
> - ❏ Accepting
>
> - ❏ Unhelpful
> - ❏ Pessimistic
> - ❏ Blaming
> - ❏ Avoidance oriented
> - ❏ Disengaged
> - ❏ Withdrawn
> - ❏ Refusing

There are many personal factors that enhance adaptive coping, which have also been found to predict resilience and PTG in many populations (Zeidner & Saklofske, 1996). These include self-awareness, self-efficacy, optimism, hope, and openness to new experiences (Calhoun & Tedeschi, 2006). These overlap the traits of emotional intelligence (EI) and effective leaders discussed earlier in the book. Coupled with our belief that leaders should have high EI and many of the factors that predict PTG, we suggest that each leader could benefit from deliberate reflection about their personal coping with the pandemic. How have you been affected by the pandemic? How have you talked with your leadership teams about what can be learned in the aftermath of crisis?

FOSTERING PTG AND RESILIENCY IN THE TEAM

Agile, resilient leaders have the responsibility to help their teams address these stresses and challenges associated with constant disruptions and uncertainty. We see this in the proliferation of acute mental healthcare services, wellness offerings, and peer support among healthcare organizations since the onset of the pandemic. Nevertheless, the burden of resilience practices cannot fall solely on individuals within the healthcare team (Cunningham, 2020). As a result of crisis leadership, opportunities for improving stronger relationships within the work environment emerge. Social support and adaptive coping via positive reappraisal are two factors attributed to resilience and PTG that can be fostered by leaders (Prati & Pietrantoni, 2009).

Previous chapters have explored the insights of our interviewed leaders related to emotional intelligence, communication, decision-making, and change, to name a few. Our open-ended questions originally did not include specific reflections or actions related to leader-facilitated coping through these unprecedented changes, yet several spoke to addressing this need in their teams. Specifically, these leaders spoke of formalized and informal means they observed, participated in, or facilitated to bolster environmental factors of social support via family and friends, camaraderie, and professional support and thereby fostering coping, resiliency, or PTG.

SOCIAL SUPPORT

In the practice environment, a sense of teamwork, perceived support, and meaning in work are all influencing factors for PTG. When traumatic experiences are related to workplace events, individual interpretation and framing, which predicts coping, will undoubtedly be influenced by their organizational experience. The degree to which an organization provides resources, encouragement, and support to role functioning is tied closely to healthcare workers' job satisfaction, fosters innovation, and improves patient satisfaction overall (Choi, 2018; Eisenberger et al., 1986; Labrague & De los Santos, 2020). Likewise, higher levels of perceived support can be protective by offsetting some stress and anxiety related to providing healthcare in times of crisis as described by these leaders.

"Leadership started to think about 'What can we do to support people's mental emotional health?' We started with leveraging relationships with community. Our community partners did wonderful things, such as donating sandwiches, cookies, and ice cream . . . it was also helping to support the local businesses."

Sharma, Director of Nursing Leadership

SOCIAL SUPPORT FROM FAMILY AND FRIENDS

"I found myself early on reaching out to people even before we got into some of the social justice issues. I was reaching out to old friends and people who had relocated, people that I hadn't talked to in a really long time again, because the relationships are important. In times like these, at least for me, it emphasized the importance of while there's work, you need relationships. Those are the things that are going to get you through the challenging work times. So, whether it's your friends, your family, or your spouse, your partners, you've got to have relationship . . . For me, it's not just about money; it's not just about work; there has to be that something else that grounds you in times of crisis."

Sharma, Director of Nursing Leadership

SOCIAL SUPPORT FROM CAMARADERIE WITH PEERS

"Listening, hearing their concerns, being available, being present . . . those were things that were incredibly important in terms of strengthening the teams caring for the healthcare workers."

Tanja, Unit Director Labor and Delivery

"I was fortunate to have been employed here for nine years, and over those nine years I feel like I've built good relationships. So, I have a strong network of support here, people that I trust. It is important to have somebody whether it's at work, at home, at church, at some sort of community or civic group . . . we need to have connections to help us through these challenging times."

Sharma, Director of Nursing Leadership

"I gave you the perspective from where I sit but our directors, nurse managers, and charge nurses have all been doing very much the same in their own units and departments. They've been working with their teams, providing huddles and food; but then there are other little things that they're doing to support the team, such as creating areas and places for rest and decompression, and being diligent about making sure teams get that break when needed so they are able to decompress."

Kathy, Chief Nursing Officer

SOCIAL SUPPORT FROM PROFESSIONAL GROUPS

"FSAP and spiritual health came up with ideas and strategies to be available to everyone. They came up with things that people could do even online in terms of wellness checks. Giving them an opportunity to voice their concerns was really impactful."

Sharma, Director of Nursing Leadership

"We had meals delivered to staff and we've partnered with our chaplains to offer time for interactions with them even while at work. We are trying to foster some sort of self-care moments as well."

Vivian, Critical Care Unit Director

"Administration developed a holistic approach that provided personal training, group exercise sessions, and yoga, offered virtually and in-person where staff were at, so it was accessible to all staff. They also had counselors, social workers, and chaplains who would lead different discussions. So, for an hour, you could come and go, but for an hour at a time, within a community virtual spot where people can join the conversation and talk about how they were going through their day, the emotional toll both personally and professionally."

Nancy, Critical Care Clinical Nurse Specialist

In crisis leadership, the goal is often restoration of normal operations/business as normal. In the aftermath of pandemic trauma, the normal must be redefined at the organizational level. PTG for teams and organizations examines a new, higher level of functioning, inclusive of lessons learned and struggles addressed. What constitutes growth among organizations will be influenced widely by workplace values and culture. It may be proactive or reactive depending on the circumstances around the trauma experience. Supportive leaders explore this, and aid in PTG for their teams by providing space for narratives, or storytelling, about how the changes have occurred and impacted operations with respect and transparency.

APPROACHES TO FOSTER ADAPTIVE COPING

Sharing lessons learned by engaging in two-way, honest reflection about difficulties and the possibilities among teams.

Mindfulness is our ability to focus on being intensely aware of what we are sensing and feeling in the moment. These practices can involve breathing methods, guided imagery, and other techniques to assist in relaxation and relief of stress.

STOP is a technique you can use to take control instead of getting caught up in a vicious cycle of worry and anxiety. Utilize these steps as a way to engage in positive actions (Mai & Davies, 2018):

S.T.O.P. is an acronym that stands for:

S — Stop, or pause

T — Take a breath

O — Observe the body, thoughts, feelings, emotions, and physical sensations

P — Proceed with more awareness

Christine Dunning (2003) describes support practices designed to provide post-trauma support to frontline workers including police officers involved in trauma on the job. Described as developing a sense of coherence, or sense-making, in the aftermath of trauma, these practices can serve a dual purpose: to enhance the likelihood of meaningful and deliberate reflection among teams and to develop trust and "being on the same page" between leadership and teams. Promoting connectedness is especially important for healthcare workers facing workplace trauma routinely (Dunning, 2003). Dunning suggests the following practices (2003):

- Establish simple rules and procedures that will be easy to grasp in the context of overwhelm.

- Respect mental models that may differ from your own and recognize how team members experience events differently.

- Recognize multiple and overlapping roles of the team as a cohesive cohort.

- Tell stories as a means of enhancing meaning-making through interaction and allow the benefit of shared experience.

- Stay connected with what Dunning calls "the field." Understanding what is happening to workers in real time allows leaders to maintain connection.

PTG is not a "Pollyanna" approach to well-being, nor does it aim to minimize the mass trauma of the healthcare workforce. Rather, PTG provides a lens to manage deliberately and actively what can emerge from this unprecedented disruption. To successfully navigate this new normal, nurse leaders will be called on to model these skills for the healthcare team in years to come. The ability to grow in the face of adversity is particularly critical for the personal well-being and career longevity of the current and incoming nursing workforce (Okoli et al., 2021). As nurse leaders explore opportunities for rebuilding workflows in the pandemic era, it will be essential that structures and processes fundamentally support the healthcare team's own agility by fostering the ability to thrive, excel, and move forward.

EXCERPT FROM "'THE PAUSE'": A DELPHI METHODOLOGY EXAMINING AN END-OF-LIFE PRACTICE"

In 2009, at a rural, Level 1 trauma center emergency department, a nurse tried something simple. He took a pause. A patient had come in by ambulance, cardiopulmonary resuscitation (CPR) was in progress, and, like 90% of patients who have CPR started in the field, this patient did not survive (Hasselqvist-Ax et al., 2015). After the attending physician pronounced the time of death, the nurse made a bold remark. He told the team to wait for a moment before moving on to the next patient. He asked them to pause and honor the life that had just ended. He asked them to consider that this patient may have had a family, that the patient loved, and the patient was loved by others. He then reminded the team that they all had tried their best to save the patient and that everyone should recognize the team's efforts. He asked for a few seconds of silence. The Pause, as a practice, is grassroots and it originated as a counter to a religious or spiritual practice in which a chaplain would be the one to ask for a moment of silence when a patient died, a moment of silence oftentimes tending toward Christian prayer (Bartels, 2014).

Reprinted with permission from Cunningham et al., 2019.

FOSTERING PTG IN ORGANIZATIONS

As you inventory possible domains of PTG for yourself, it is natural to contemplate your organization's progress. Similar to re-envisioning the strategic operations systems and communication portions of the emergency response plan based on key learnings during the pandemic, perhaps there is an opportunity to re-imagine employer commitment to employee well-being, stress response, and coping. Foremost, the leadership team must answer the direct question: Does the employer have an obligation to tend to the critical psychological stress needs of employees exposed to trauma while delivering healthcare? Does attending to the well-being of healthcare workers fall within the mission, vision, and values of the organization? If so, does the leadership team have the knowledge, resources, and ability to develop such a crisis response plan, engage the necessary personnel, and provide learning opportunities to mitigate the situation? A leader-engaged approach to fostering PTG is fundamental to growth among teams facing pervasive, chronic trauma in the workplace, and it begins with transparent discussions/questions like these (see Table 9.4).

TABLE 9.4 Posttraumatic Growth–Informed Approaches for Leaders and Organizations

Leaders	Organizations
Effective, transparent communication	Provide resilience-oriented interventions at all levels
Learn to recognize your own distressing thoughts and emotions	Provide leaders with resources needed for supportive work environments among teams
Guide teams in perceiving the opportunity for transformation and change	Remain open to opportunity for growth, innovation, creativity arising from crisis
Create spaces for listening and sharing of experiences	Prioritize deliberate reflection and emotional support among leadership

At one of the large hospital systems, this has become a pressing issue for the leadership team, resulting in the creation of a Co-Chief Well-Being Officer position, assumed by the Vice President of Practice and Innovation. Additionally, Michelle, the Innovation and Advancement Coordinator, recognized the need to nurture her team and employ proven tactics for fostering coping:

"I'm very involved with work on resiliency and the Community Resiliency Model (CRM). I was able to undertake the training and have now been co-teaching CRM since before the pandemic started. Recognizing the huge need for this training in our nursing and frontline staff, we tried to teach the important elements of resiliency but shorten the class . . . What we were trying to convey to staff and our bedside nurses is you're going to have to try to find something that will help you manage this stress. So, we taught small portions of the CRM and wellness among staff."

Michelle, Innovation and Advancement Coordinator

This commitment of the hospital to mental health and well-being for all is a fundamental change in priorities from years past and falls in lines with organizational PTG. Perhaps the culture would have eventually led to the recognition for specific wellness positions and to the develop of a comprehensive wellness plan, but most certainly the pandemic elevated the necessity. From here, much work is needed to quantify progress, develop sustainable plans, and measure results. We anticipate this investment will be justified by retaining more fulfilled, perhaps even more resilient or matured, employees and leaders. At this juncture, having weathered the challenges of a pandemic that shook the foundation of our nursing profession as evidenced by the massive exodus of nurses, employers are not going to successfully retain them with raising salaries alone. Certainly, the literally life-saving work nurses perform daily and in extreme conditions deserves appropriate recognition and compensation that is perhaps long overdue, but this strategy alone does not address the core need of personal well-being. Ultimately, compensation and recognition without addressing individual welfare will not end the revolving mass-exodus door and allow for team cohesion, excellence in patient outcomes, and employee satisfaction.

COMMUNITY RESILIENCY MODEL

The Community Resiliency Model (CRM) is a skills-based stabilization program that teaches community members to help themselves and others through simple interventions based on cutting edge research about the brain. One of CRM's key objectives is to expand access to biologically based treatments by training frontline service providers, community leaders, and clinicians. The goal is to help create "trauma-informed" and "resiliency-focused" communities that share a common understanding of the impact of trauma and chronic stress on the nervous system and how resiliency can be restored.

For more information and to find a training program near you, see https://www.traumaresourceinstitute.com/crm.

KEY TAKEAWAYS

Acknowledging the acute (now chronic) stress of the pandemic's toll on our healthcare systems is evident across every aspect of our daily lives and threatens the very structure of our national and global healthcare systems. This pandemic, and its wake of social, political, and economic damage, calls on us to ask, "What good can possibly come of this?" In the face of such ongoing tragedy, stress, and strain, sometimes it can be hard to know the next right step for leaders navigating the unknown alongside the suffering of their teams. Employing measures and interventions to foster resiliency, coping, and PTG within ourselves, employees, and organizations is a critical step to providing a safe and compassionate worksite. Incorporating a commitment to employee wellness within the mission, vision, and values of an organization is the transformational change in PTG which must guide decisions as healthcare entities rebuild.

A commitment to wellness as an organizational value is a requirement in fostering health and addressing the hybrid disaster that started with a pandemic but has now culminated into a desperate nursing shortage.

Numerous opportunities exist for inclusion of well-being into the workplace such as ongoing screening, similar to an annual physical, to assess employment of techniques described in this chapter from the Posttraumatic Growth Inventory, enhancing access to mental health professionals, and acknowledging and rewarding excellence in the team. These will be just a few of the suggestions we'll tackle in our final chapter on application and moving forward. When asked about his hopes for Covid recovery and moving forward, Carson, Vice President of Nursing Practice and Education, replied:

> "My hope is that we don't go back to our old ways. I hope we don't have refractory leadership when things slow down. I hope we as leaders have that ability to self-assess without rose-colored lenses and retain the great things that should be kept: huddles at a regular cadence with teams; greater interprofessional communication; authentic acknowledgment; talking more about DEI; and attention to resilience and well-being. These have been brought to [the] table. Now we need to move from the talk and surface to doing the deep work."
>
> Carson, Vice President of Nursing Practice and Education

REFLECTIVE EXERCISES

9.1 → DELIBERATE REFLECTION

Consider how the pandemic or another crisis has directly affected you.

Describe one particular difficulty

What were your three biggest concerns?
1.

2.

3.

How did you handle each concern? Who or what helped you get through it?
1.

2.

3.

How do you view this situation now?

9.2 → IDENTIFYING INDIVIDUAL AND ORGANIZATIONAL AREAS OF PTG

Reflect on the guiding questions in Table 9.3, contemplate PTG growth you personally have experienced during the past two years. What evolution have you witnessed or contributed to within the organization?

Individual	Organizational

9.3 → RESILIENCY

Is resiliency a trait or a skill?

Can resiliency be fostered in others?

Is there a corporate responsibility to foster resiliency in employees?

Describe specific actions you could take to foster resiliency in your team.

REFERENCES

American Psychiatric Association. (2013). *Diagnostic and statistical manual of mental disorders* (5th ed.). American Psychiatric Publishing.

American Psychological Association. (2022a). *Coping*. https://dictionary.apa.org/coping

American Psychological Association. (2022b). *Trauma*. https://www.apa.org/topics/trauma

Calhoun, L. G., & Tedeschi, R. G. (Eds.). (2006). *Handbook of posttraumatic growth: Research and practice*. Lawrence Erlbaum Associates.

Choi, B. S. (2018). Influence of social support and resilience on the nurse job performance. *Indian Journal of Public Health Research & Development, 9*(3), 788–792. https://doi.org/10.1177/0193945916685712

Cunningham, T. (2020). The burden of resilience should not fall solely on nurses. *American Journal of Nursing, 120*(9), 11. https://doi.org/10.1097/01.NAJ.0000697544.96740.a6

Cunningham, T., Ducar, D. M., & Keim-Malpass, J. (2019). "The Pause": A Delphi methodology examining an end-of-life practice. *Western Journal of Nursing Research, 41*(10), 1481–1498. https://doi.org/10.1177/0193945919826314

Cunningham, T., & Pfeiffer, K. (2022). Posttraumatic growth as a model to measure and guide implementation of COVID-19 recovery and resiliency. *Nursing Administration Quarterly, 46*(1), 81–87. https://doi.org/10.1097/NAQ.0000000000000509

Dunning, C. (2003). Sense of coherence in managing trauma workers. In D. Paton, J. M. Violanti, & L. M. Smith (Eds.), *Promoting capabilities to manage posttraumatic stress: Perspectives on resilience* (Chapter 9). Charles C. Thomas.

Eisenberger, R., Huntington, R., Hutchison, S., & Sowa, D. (1986). Perceived organizational support. *Journal of Applied Psychology, 71*(3), 500–507.

Finstad, G. L., Giorgi, G., Lulli, L. G., Pandolfi, C., Foti, G., León-Perez, J. M., Cantero-Sánchez, F. J., & Mucci, N. (2021). Resilience, coping strategies and posttraumatic growth in the workplace following COVID-19: A narrative review on the positive aspects of trauma. *International Journal of Environmental Research and Public Health, 18*(18), 9453. https://doi.org/10.3390/ijerph18189453

Folkman, S., & Moskowitz, J. T. (2004). Coping: Pitfalls and promise. *Annual Review of Psychology, 55*, 745–774. https://doi.org/10.1146/annurev.psych.55.090902.141456

Haas, M. (2015). *Bouncing forward: Transforming bad breaks into breakthroughs*. Enliven.

Higgins, T. (2020, March 27). Coronavirus pandemic could inflict emotional trauma and PTSD on an unprecedented scale scientists warn. *CNBC*. https://www.cnbc.com/2020/03/27/coronavirus-pandemic-could-inflict-long-lasting-emotional-trauma-ptsd.html

Hill, E. M., & Watkins, K. (2017). Women with ovarian cancer: Examining the role of social support and rumination in posttraumatic growth, psychological distress, and psychological well-being. *Journal of Clinical Psychology in Medical Settings, 24*(1), 47–58. https://doi.org/10.1007/s10880-016-9482-7

Hirooka, K., Fukahori, H., Taku, K., Togari, T., & Ogawa, A. (2017). Quality of death, rumination, and posttraumatic growth among bereaved family members of cancer patients in home palliative care. *Psycho-Oncology, 26*(12), 2168–2174. https://doi.org/10.1002/pon.4446

International Council of Nurses. (2021a, January 13). *The COVID-19 effect: World's nurses facing mass trauma, an immediate danger to the profession and future of our health systems*. https://www.icn.ch/news/covid-19-effect-worlds-nurses-facing-mass-trauma-immediate-danger-profession-and-future-our

International Council of Nurses. (2021b, October 21). *ICN says 115,000 healthcare worker deaths from COVID-19 exposes collective failure of leaders to protect global workforce*. https://www.icn.ch/news/icn-says-115000-healthcare-worker-deaths-covid-19-exposes-collective-failure-leaders-protect

Janoff-Bulman, R. (1989). Assumptive worlds and the stress of traumatic events: Applications of the schema construct. *Social Cognition, 7*(2), 113–136. https://doi.org/10.1521/soco.1989.7.2.113

Labrague, L. J., & De los Santos, J. (2020). COVID-19 anxiety among front-line nurses: Predictive role of organisational support, personal resilience and social support. *Journal of Nursing Management, 28*(7), 1653–1661. https://doi.org/10.1111/jonm.13121

Lazarus, R. S., & Folkman, S. (1984). *Stress, appraisal, and coping*. Springer Publishing Company.

Leys, C., Arnal, C., Wollast, R., Rolin, H., Kotsou, I., & Fossion, P. (2020). Perspectives on resilience: Personality trait or skill? *European Journal of Trauma & Dissociation, 4*(2), 1–6.

Luthar, S. S., Cicchetti, D., & Becker, B. (2000). The construct of resilience: A critical evaluation and guidelines for future work. *Child Development, 71*(3), 543–562. https://doi.org/10.1111/1467-8624.00164

Mai, T., & Davies, R. (2018, September 20). Practice: S.T.O.P. *Accelerate Learning Community*. https://accelerate.uofuhealth.utah.edu/resilience/practice-s-t-o-p

Maitlis, S. (2020). Posttraumatic growth at work. *Annual Review of Organizational Psychology and Organizational Behavior, 7*(1), 395–419. https://doi.org/10.1146/annurev-orgpsych-012119-044932

Nurse.org. (2022). *This is the state of nursing.* https://media.nurse.org/docs/State+of+Nursing+-+2022.pdf

Okoli, C. T. C., Seng, S., Lykins, A., & Higgins, J. T. (2021). Correlates of post-traumatic growth among nursing professionals: A cross-sectional analysis. *Journal of Nursing Management, 29,* 307– 316. https://doi.org/10.1111/jonm.13155

Olson, K., Shanafelt, T., & Southwick, S. (2020). Pandemic-driven posttraumatic growth for organizations and individuals. *JAMA, 324*(18), 1829–1830. https://doi.org/10.1001/jama.2020.20275

Prati, G., & Pietrantoni, L. (2009). Optimism, social support, and coping strategies as factors contributing to posttraumatic growth: A meta-analysis. *Journal of Loss and Trauma, 14,* 364–288. https://doi.org/10.1080/15325020902724271

Rutter, M. (1985). Resilience in the face of adversity: Protective factors and resistance to psychiatric disorder. *British Journal of Psychiatry, 147*(6), 598–611. https://doi.org/10.1192/bjp.147.6.598

Schaefer, J. A., & Moos, R. H. (1992). Life crises and personal growth. In B. N. Carpenter (Ed.), *Personal coping: Theory, research, and application* (pp. 149–170). Praeger Publishers/Greenwood Publishing Group.

Schubert, C. F., Schmidt, U., & Rosner, R. (2016). Posttraumatic growth in populations with posttraumatic stress disorder – A systematic review on growth-related psychological constructs and biological variables. *Clinical Psychology & Psychotherapy, 23*(6), 469–486. https://doi.org/10.1002/cpp.1985

Stockton, H., Hunt, N., & Joseph, S. (2011). Cognitive processing, rumination, and posttraumatic growth. *Journal of Traumatic Stress, 24*(1), 85–92. https://doi.org/10.1002/jts.20606

Tedeschi, R. G., & Calhoun, L. (1995). *Trauma & transformation: Growing in the aftermath of suffering.* Sage Publications.

Tedeschi, R. G., Shakespeare-Finch, J., Taku, K., & Calhoun, L. G. (2018). *Posttraumatic growth: Theory, research, and applications.* Routledge, Taylor & Francis Group.

Zeidner, M., & Saklofske, D. (1996). Adaptive and maladaptive coping. In M. Zeidner & N. S. Endler (Eds.), *Handbook of coping: Theory, research, applications* (pp. 505–531). John Wiley & Sons.

Zoellner, T., & Maercker, A. (2006). Posttraumatic growth in clinical psychology – A critical review and introduction of a two component model. *Clinical Psychology Review, 26*(5), 626–653. https://doi.org/10.1016/j.cpr.2006.01.008

"This is not the end. It is not even the beginning of the end. But it is, perhaps, the end of the beginning."
—**Winston Churchill**

10

New Beginnings

In thinking about concluding something in our lives, as humans we like to reflect on what we've learned and how we would approach things differently with the experience we now have.

Similarly, in combing through the transcripts, we noted that our various leaders referred to "lessons learned" 33 times, primarily centering around the need for better preparation, communication, and emotional support for themselves and their team.

> **WE ASKED NURSE LEADERS**
>
> → What did you learn?
>
> → What could you have done better?
>
> → If given the opportunity, what would you do over?

"I think one big lesson that we've learned is that communication is key . . . without communication nothing happens, and consistent regular detailed communication has been very important for us, as leaders."

Carson, Vice President of Nursing Practice and Education

"We learned we had to shore up some structures of communications between the entities. With supplies, we really had to work together due to big supply shortages. I don't know if there will be specific training required for the future, but I think that there have been some systems that have been impacted by this, that are now seen as a silver lining. We've made changes and we're not going to go back to the old way."

Tanja, Unit Director Labor and Delivery

"I've learned that you definitely need someone in place that can guide staff through things like this. Someone that's well-informed, visible, present, calm, because your staff are going to need that support . . . I don't care how much training you give them. I realized the true situation when that first patient came in, and the level of anxiety that was in the unit that day. I don't think I've ever seen that in all my years."

Symone, Education Coordinator for NICU

"I learned to have a mindset for the long term, pulling your team in close and quick."

Nancy, Critical Care Clinical Nurse Specialist

"We need to be better prepared. I would say maybe we could do some drills from an infection prevention side of things, maybe annually or bi-annually for our leadership teams on how we respond to pandemics. How can we get our staff on board just like we do fire drills and other emergencies? I think having drills in place for these types of things would be key for how we handle things in the future."

Symone, Education Coordinator for NICU

"I realized I needed to have breathing space; taking the time to recognize that you are also stressed. And that that's OK; that's part of a normal process. You don't have to fight against that. But really, it's about the recognition, and taking the time that you need in order to fill yourself back up."

Vivian, Critical Care Unit Director

In Chapters 7 and 8, we discussed principles for incident command and standardized communication, referencing NIMS training and CDC documents for assuring hospital preparedness. Recently, the Department of Health and Human Services Assistant Secretary for Assistance and Response released a Technical Resources, Assistance Center, and Information Exchange (TRACIE) tip sheet highlighting several key observations about how healthcare ICS functioned during the Covid-19 pandemic, including lessons learned collected from interviews, surveys, and literature reviews as of August 2021. An electronic copy can be found at https://files.asprtracie.hhs.gov/documents/aspr-tracie-the-effect-of-covid-19-on-the-healthcare-ics.pdf.

Validating many of our findings, this tip sheet supports the clear delineation of roles and responsibilities using the ICS structure. It supports implementing strong communication strategies, integrating clinical personnel in the ICS process and decision-making, alternative care delivery strategies such as telemedicine, and recognizing the need for team support and strategies for promoting resiliency and well-being.

THE WAVE MINDSET

One particular aspect of this report that we support is to embrace a "wave" mindset. As discussed by our leaders, Covid surges came in waves that were massive tsunamis but then were followed by some calmer seas. Our leaders found that time between "waves" allowed for three valuable insights: 1. Mental and physical reset; 2. Reflection and re-evaluation; and 3. Opportunity to change roles.

MENTAL AND PHYSICAL RESET

Foremost is that the time between waves allowed for a period of mental and physical reset. Leaders and team members alike were encouraged to utilize their days off and recharge, as described by Tanja, Unit Director Labor and Delivery:

> "I'm lucky to have a leader that was also really focused on making sure we took care of ourselves and making us take time off. Because we were also coming in on the weekends to round on the weekend staff, we were taking turns doing that. She was really intentional: 'By the end of this week, I need you to find some days that you're going to take off and let me know what they are.'"
>
> Tanja, Unit Director Labor and Delivery

REFLECTION AND RE-EVALUATION

Secondly, the waves allowed for a clear re-evaluation time. As supported by the TRACIE tip sheet, ongoing performance improvement is critical, with the evaluation and then re-evaluation of processes implemented. One suggestion is to implement a "wave" After Action Report approach, where the incident scope period for a report is redefined as the beginning and end of a given "wave" or surge period. Time and again, we heard from our leaders that processes put into place during the first wave were re-evaluated and refined for the second and then third waves. Some reflected that a more formalized process of data collection and refinement would have better facilitated rapid response:

> "Following the first wave, when I looked at a performance evaluation, I saw that there was a very siloed leadership in our hospital system. Why couldn't we have done things all together at the same time versus having to reinvent the wheel every single time? Additionally, no matter what type of decision you make, there are always unintended consequences to that decision. And a lot of times what you have to do is just go with that decision and then deal with the unintended consequences. I felt like there were missed opportunities for us for data collection in our response."
>
> Kimberly, Nurse Anesthetist and Nursing Faculty

OPPORTUNITY TO CHANGE ROLES

Finally, having a "wave mindset" allows for the opportunity to change roles and leadership. In some cases, this may be the actual people assigned to the various roles of Incident Commander or Logistics Leader, or simply an opportunity to change a leadership approach to a situation.

Having time for a reset, even a mental reset, after reflection over the process and outcomes allows for a new beginning. This allowance for a reset during the break in the waves requires transparency and dialogue. It requires the honest appraisal as a team of what went well, what was disastrous, and how changes can be enacted. With a wave mindset during a crisis, resetting leadership is not a termination, but instead an opportunity to foster new growth, an allowance for grace and appreciation, and refinement to maximize effectiveness. Sometimes the most effective, visionary CEO during a period of growth is not the most effective Incident Commander during crisis, but their leadership and role within the organization is still necessary, just not as the Incident Commander.

This acceptance of changing of roles and leadership priorities as part of a wave mentality was articulated after the second wave by Andrew, Chief Quality Officer in Nursing. Note his recognition of the temporal situation that inevitably will change:

> "I would say now, it's a little more back to normal now with my role than it was. I think that's because we don't have as many, at least as of right now, we don't have as many urgent initiatives as we did right in the beginning. So we've gone back, the role has changed from starting up a whole bunch of new policy, new process, new protocols, to figuring out how do we still do all of our normal work in the presence of Covid. In the future, we're going to have more Covid surges, I think it's inevitable. But we can't, as an organization, just shut down. We're going to have to figure out how we tackle the increased volume and at the same time, figure out how to keep our surgeries going, our ambulatory visits going and promote televisits. Also, to figure out ways to keep the IT work going for the care of cardiac patients or the care of transplant patients who still need care. I think that's where it has shifted a little bit, is trying to figure out how to balance both. But I'd say that my work is a little more back to normal now than it was. We'll see if that changes with a third surge or not."

> Andrew, Chief Quality Officer in Nursing

THE SECONDARY CRISIS: THE NURSING SHORTAGE

As this book was being written, we made note of the secondary crisis of the nursing shortage that was developing over the Covid pandemic crisis. A Google search today of "nursing shortage Covid" returns no less than 7,520,000 results from news articles, scholarly research, and opinions. Lots of opinions. For "physician shortage Covid," the return is about half as much at 4,590,000. Yet this is not the priority of the public who would more fiercely debate "vaccine mandate" (generating 288,000,000 hits) than recognize that the lack of healthcare providers will likely more directly affect their health than a vaccination against the pandemic that exacerbated this workforce shortage.

The literature over the past 30 years supports that staffing ratios directly impact outcomes of morbidity and mortality (Aiken et al., 2002; Griffiths et al., 2019; Needleman et al., 2011). Specifically, every extra patient on a nurse's caseload increased mortality rates by 7%, often due to care left undone or inability to directly observe and catch patient deterioration due to the high number of patients (Aiken et al., 2002). In other studies, higher patient ratios have been associated with higher rates of nosocomial infections in hospitalized patients (Cho et al., 2003; Kovner et al., 2000, 2002; Needleman et al., 2002). Still additional studies have documented increased lengths of stay with high patient to nurse ratios (Lichtig et al., 1999; Pronovost et al., 1999). Finally, a study from Queensland, New Zealand published during the pandemic found that minimum nurse-to-patient mandates were associated with reductions in 30-day mortality, greater reductions in length of stay, and significant cost savings in hospitals with mandated staffing ratios compared to those without (McHugh et al., 2021).

Wading into the debates of mandated nurse to patient ratios is beyond the scope and intent of this book about leadership during a crisis, but we cannot ignore that nursing leadership will be inextricably involved in addressing nurse workforce burnout and shortage. Recognizing the toll of the Covid pandemic on nurse leaders in particular, the American Organization for Nursing Leadership (AONL) and Joslin Marketing partnered to conduct a longitudinal study on nurse leaders' primary challenges, staffing shortages, and nurse leader well-being (AONL, 2021).

This longitudinal online survey was first launched in July of 2020 with 1,824 leaders completing or partially completing that survey, followed by a second survey in February 2021 completed by 2,741 nurse leaders, and finally a third survey completed by 1,781 nurse leaders in August 2021. Most of the respondents identified as Caucasian, were over the age of 45, and from urban acute care hospitals. Eighty percent were either chief nursing officers, chief nursing executives (CNO/CNE), vice presidents, directors, or managers.

Most notable changes in the types of concerns from the first to the last survey were a decrease in concerns regarding adequate supplies and PPE, and the communication and implementation of policy changes. Replacing these concerns has been the emotional health and well-being of nursing staff, coupled with staff retention.

Sadly, the AONL released findings from this longitudinal study of nurse leaders in August of 2021 in which 25% of nurse leaders reported they were not emotionally healthy. Another 32% reported being neutral on this question while just 43% reported feeling emotionally or very emotionally healthy. This is coupled with a noted data trend that more nurse leaders report considering leaving their current role from the first to the most recent survey point, with a full 17% of nurse leaders now saying they are considering leaving. Perhaps driving this dissatisfaction with their present position is the fact that 90% of nurse leaders most recently surveyed believe their organizations will experience a nurse staffing shortage post pandemic. To address this, thus far, 76% of their organizations increased wages, bonuses, or incentives; 56% have increased or added float pools; and a full third are considering supplementing staffing arrangements to include team-based nursing with assistive personnel. Sadly, nurse leader confidence in their teams' ability to handle the next surge or pandemic was noted to drop sharply to just a 57% confidence level (AONL, 2021).

A NEW NURSING LEADERSHIP

Clearly both the professional nurses directly working in patient care and their leaders are battle worn. Yet, we know the enduring, resilient spirit of nurses. For every time a nurse feels defeated, crumples with weariness and the emotional distress from not being able to do enough, they return the next day to care again. This is the essence of nursing as the most trusted profession. For the 20th straight year running per the 2022 Gallup poll, nurses are the most trusted professionals with an 81% approval rating from the public (Saad, 2022). This far exceeds even the second-place profession, medical doctors at 67%, grade-school teachers at 64%, pharmacists at 63%, and military officers at 61%. Americans view nurses as highly ethical, and coming out the other side of Covid, we believe despite the weariness and internal struggles the profession is enduring, it will grow stronger.

In fact, while nursing remains the essence of caring, a new persona is also emerging for the profession. Nurses are emerging as leaders in their own right; leaders because they are centered on self and others. In the foreword of a newly released book, *Human-Centered Leadership in Healthcare: Evolution of a Revolution,* Dr. Jean Watson asserts that "Leadership is and cannot be otherwise—Human-Centered"(p. xviii). In work begun before the Covid pandemic, authors Leclerc et al. (2022) share their expert knowledge, vision, and grounded research to propose a new framework for leadership in healthcare that is fundamental to the daily actions and beliefs of nurses. In reflection, many of the leadership theories recited within this book up until this point have been borrowed from business. Many of the quotes that started off each chapter or section were borrowed from politicians, entrepreneurs, industrial giants, and entertainers, yet the meat of our story is reflection from nurse leaders in the ICUs, in the nurseries, assisting a laboring woman, and in the Incident Command System that reflect that nursing leadership is centered on the humanity of their teams.

As we wrap up this book, we encourage you to consider a deep dive into Human-Centered Leadership. Adhering to systematic and rigorous qualitative methodology based on constructivist grounded theory, Leclerc et al. (2021) conducted extensive focus groups with 35 nurses and leaders from across healthcare. The purpose of their research was to explore and explain how nurses and nurse leaders respond to and navigate the landscape of caring for complex humans within an industry that is focused on efficiency and profitability. Their interviews centered on two simple questions: "How would you describe the nurse leader you would follow to the ends of the earth?" and "How would you describe the nurse leader who made you consider leaving your job?" From extensive recordings, 15 thematic attributes resulted, which the authors then mapped into three dimensions that personify the Human-Centered Leader: the Awakener, the Connector, and the Upholder as seen in Figure 10.1.

This visual framework depicts an approach to leadership that starts with the leader at center, who uses their mind, body, and spirit to influence the environment around them. This leader understands that they have the ability to influence and innovate; they have the ability to create a culture of trust, a culture of caring, and a culture of excellence. Because the leader has this influence, they must be aware of and also foster self-care and self-compassion through mindfulness and well-being. By caring for self first, the leader develops and sustains the capacity to care for others. From this central core, the authors assert that human-centered leaders then connect central leadership attributes of the Awakener, the Connector, and the Upholder to cultures of Excellence, Trust, and Caring (see Figure 10.1). Each effective leader has these attributes within them, though they may naturally express one more strongly than the others. The authors provide multiple examples of each dimension's attributes, exemplars, and practical measures to enhance and develop skills.

THE AWAKENER

The Awakener is focused on developing others. Natural teachers, Awakeners are focused on cultivating people. Their drive is to deliver great results (supporting a culture of excellence) by developing their workforce. Their motivation is intrinsic as they connect their team by being the coach, the mentor, the advocate, and even the architect that designs structure for team growth. These leaders highly value many of the shared leadership and shared governance approaches previously discussed in this book.

THE CONNECTOR

The Connector unites the team around the common vision, values, and mission. This dimension is focused on uniting the community and creating a healthy work environment through collaboration, offering support, embracing experimentation and innovation, and fostering authentic communication. Efforts here result in a culture of trust with team members engaged in the work.

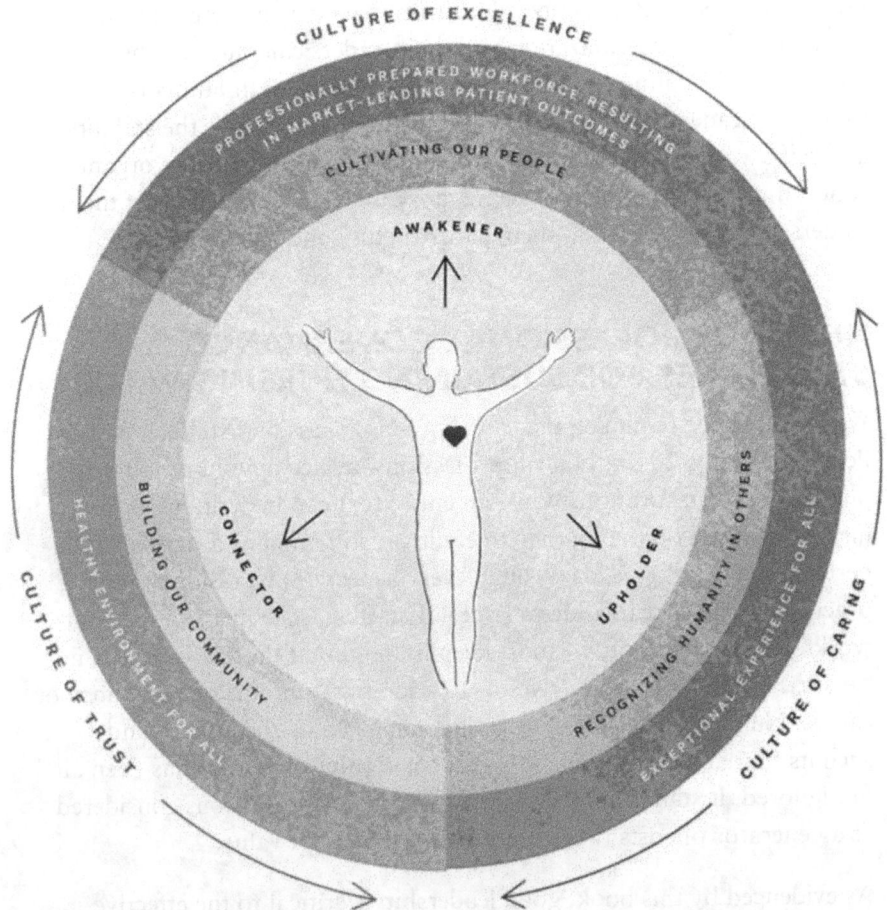

FIGURE 10.1 Human-Centered Leadership Model.
Note: Reprinted with permission from Lucy LeClerc.

THE UPHOLDER

The Upholder is focused on that one-to-one relationship; is emotionally, socially, and organizationally aware; and demonstrates respect, kindness, empathy, and empowerment. The leader, mindful of the Upholder dimension, models self-care and encourages it in their team.

We applaud this model as it conceptualizes the essence and observations we gleaned through our qualitative interviews, thematic analysis, and exploration of crisis leadership found within these pages. While completed independently, our work validates and nicely complements the

Human-Centered Leadership in Healthcare Model and returns us to a solid tenet that an organization and their leaders can only weather a crisis when the culture is built on a solid foundation. In Human-Centered Leadership in Healthcare, the core foundation is the stability and self-awareness of the leader. Similarly, a strong healthcare organization must invest in the well-being, growth, and development of their leaders as richly as they do their infrastructure and technology.

NURSING PROFESSIONAL GOVERNANCE: STRUCTURES FOR SUSTAINING NURSING VALUE

We must also be reminded that nursing is a profession (Malloch & Porter-O'Grady, 2019). Like all professions, its accountability is to the public, not the institution. While an entire text can be written on the historic struggle on the journey to equity, it still remains a significant underlying issue that threads through every aspect of professional nursing practice. While we can address issues of staffing, schedules, ratios, and workload management, we must keep in mind that those are effects, not causes. Focusing on them drives us to address symptoms rather than root causes. Nursing has historically been managed as a cost center, and as such its fundamental value and impact as a value generator has been all but ignored. It stands alone among all the major professions considered as a generator of costs rather than as a producer of value.

As evidenced by this book, good leadership is critical to the effective management of crisis and the support of nursing practice and practitioners in it. It must be remembered, however, that behavior cannot be sustained unless the prevailing structures support it (Albert et al., 2021). In fact, the structure supporting nursing practice provides the framework that determines what form that practice will take. This is no less true in a crisis. In fact, in many of the post-pandemic surveys of nurses, many shared how both the structures influencing decision-making—including incident command—reduced or eliminated the practicing nurses' engagement, inclusion, and participation in those decisions that affected nursing practice. It was this, many claimed, that led to feelings of disenfranchisement, disengagement, and dissatisfaction (Robbins & Lesser, 2022). Failing to fully utilize nursing professional governance structures or abandoning them altogether was also identified as a contributing factor to nurses' feelings of loss (ANA Enterprise, n.d.).

Professions govern their practice (Clavelle et al., 2016). Structures that enable this demonstrate ownership of the accountabilities related to practice, quality, competence, and their body of knowledge. Structures of professional governance assure that nurses maintain this accountability and participation in its exercise as a fundamental expectation of their membership in the professional community. These professional governance structures also assure the engagement and contribution of practicing nurses in decisions and actions that affect the defining relationship between nurse and patient.

Part of the work of reconstructing the nursing culture in healthcare organizations going forward will include an assessment of the mechanisms of decision-making and the organizational structures and behaviors that are the essential levers for facilitating nurse engagement in decisions, actions, and evaluations that affect their capacity for excellence in nursing practice. Re-enabling nursing professional governance structures can further establish strong accountability and ownership for nursing practice, acting as a driver for both determining and advancing nursing value.

CHANGE FOR THE BETTER

Despite the trauma and losses, we have witnessed some changes that may improve healthcare, and nursing directly. Most assuredly, one of the most public changes has been the rapid uptake and continued use of telemedicine. As explained by Dr. Shantanu Nundy in his recent book, *Care After Covid: What the Pandemic Revealed Is Broken in Healthcare and How to Reinvent It* (2021), healthcare is now meeting patients where they are in the community, at home, and on their devices. This allows healthcare providers to connect with patients in new ways. He specifically encourages "distributed care," where care happens not in clinics and hospitals, but in homes and the community, and "digitally enabled care," in which providers are directly interacting with patients to monitor progress via apps and frequent, short telehealth check-ins.

For nursing, one of the most notable changes during the pandemic was the relaxation of state regulations for licensure. Within weeks of the first patient being diagnosed in the US, every state had declared a state of emergency allowing nurses licensed in other states to receive rapid processing of licenses (National Council of State Boards of Nursing

[NCSBN], 2020). While some of these statutes have expired, this certainly brought into focus the need for enhanced nursing compact licensure. As of January 2022, 33 states have enacted and implemented a nursing license compact with updated information readily available at https://www.ncsbn.org/compacts.htm. The Nurse Licensure Compact (NLC) allows a nurse to have one multistate license with the ability to practice in the home state and other compact states. In hindsight, if all states had been part of the NLC prior to Covid-19, nurses could have easily mobilized to areas of highest need, such as Seattle and New York City. More information about current state licensure rules and emergency rulings can be found at https://www.ncsbn.org/news/covid19/emergency-response-by-states-and-nurses.page

Within nursing education, most classes and clinicals have resumed, and the modifications to the NCLEX put into place during the first few months of the Covid pandemic expired on September 30, 2020 (NCSBN, n.d.). Presently, the 2019 NCLEX-RN test plan remains in effect until the new NextGen examination begins in Spring of 2023. This NCLEX-RN is a variable length, computerized adaptive test and can range from 75–145 items, provided with a time limit of five hours (https://www.ncsbn.org/testplans.htm).

Success over the past year in replacing some clinical rotations with simulations and replacing in-person instruction with online and distance education has allowed for the exploration of alternative educational deliveries and permanent reconfiguring of programs. For the self-motivated and disciplined student, quality asynchronous programs offer a means for nurses to advance their education at a pace and delivery that may work better for them. However, in a recent study by Michel et al. (2021), 772 nursing prelicensure students who participated in a mixed methods study exploring their perceptions about the pandemic's effects on their education and intention to join the nursing workforce disagreed. In general, they noted barriers to online learning forced by the pandemic and felt less engaged with their education, experienced a lack of communication from faculty, increased workloads, social and academic isolation, and anxiety about learning. These students were concerned about their lack of in-person clinical experiences and felt they may not have the requisite knowledge to enter the workforce; however, the vast majority still planned to enter into it.

Our final observation for the better centers around nurses becoming more publicly involved, engaged, and visible. Yes, nurses are loved and trusted by the public. But the reality is that nurses have been an invisible workforce, the largest segment of the healthcare workforce, but with virtually no presence in the media. A study from George Washington University in 2017 found that nurses were featured as a source in just 2% of healthcare information, down from 4% 20 years prior (Mason et al., 2018). The lead author of that study wrote a compelling editorial in *USA Today* in June of 2020 lamenting the great contributions of nurses coupled with the lack of recognition and the lack of representation by nurses in the media and on hospital boards (Mason, 2020).

A recent opinion piece from England (Garcia & Qureshi, 2022) made similar observations about the unexpected media attention now paid to nurses during the pandemic, including the negative stereotyping of female nurses, the media's explicit negative messaging surrounding male and ethnic nurses, and finally the deprofessionalizing of nursing as a vocation. We close this book with an acknowledgment that all professional nurses must be seen, must be heard, and must be appreciated. As nursing leaders, we must now pick up one more mantle and advocate for them; advocate for adequate staffing, for adequate compensation, for equal representation in the board rooms and arenas where patient care decisions are made. As leaders emerging from a crisis, we must call attention to the contributions of nurses at every level and work beside our educators, legislature, and mainstream media to reinvent the image of nurses to accurately portray who our nurses are, their educational preparation, their skills, and the lives they impact.

In this post-pandemic period, there is much opportunity for reflection on leader experiences inside a crisis that will continue to inform the development and maturation of nurse leaders. The healthcare system's corrections and transformations will accelerate, driven by insight and learning from pandemic leader experiences and challenges. The editors hope that this text serves as a window into these leaders' observations and experiences and accelerates dialogue and development that will inform their continuing growth and effectiveness. The journey continues, and so does the hope that nursing leaders will advance their scholarship and practice excellence as the healthcare system evolves to higher levels of effectiveness and positive impact for all whom nurses serve.

REFERENCES

Aiken, L. H., Clarke, S. P., Sloane, D. M., Sochalski, J., & Silber, J. H. (2002). Hospital nurse staffing and patient mortality, nurse burnout, and job dissatisfaction. *JAMA, 288*(16), 1987–1993. https://doi.org/10.1001/jama.288.16.1987

Albert, N., Pappas, S., Porter-O'Grady, T., & Malloch, K. (2021). *Quantum leadership: Creating sustainable value in healthcare* (6th ed.). Jones & Bartlett.

American Organization of Nursing Leadership. (2021). *COVID-19 longitudinal study August 2021 report: Nurse leaders' top challenges, emotional health, and areas of need support, July 2020 to August 2021.* https://www.aonl.org/system/files/media/file/2021/09/AONL%20COVID-19%20Longitudinal%203%20Written%20Report.pdf

ANA Enterprise. (n.d.). *COVID-19 survey series results.* https://www.nursingworld.org/practice-policy/work-environment/health-safety/disaster-preparedness/coronavirus/what-you-need-to-know/survey-series-results/

Cho, S. H., Ketefian, S., Barkauskas, V. H., & Smith, D. G. (2003). The effects of nurse staffing on adverse events, morbidity, mortality, and medical costs. *Nursing Research, 52*(2), 71–79. https://doi.org/10.1097/00006199-200303000-00003

Clavelle, J., Porter-O'Grady, T., Weston, M., & Veran, J. (2016). Evolution of structural empowerment: Moving from shared to professional governance. *Journal of Nursing Administration, 46*(6), 308–312.

Garcia, R., & Qureshi, I. (2022). Nurse identity: Reality and media portrayal. *Evidence-Based Nursing, 25*(1), 1–5. https://doi.org/10.1136/ebnurs-2021-103480

Griffiths, P., Maruotti, A., Recio Saucedo, A., Redfern, O. C., Ball, J. E., Briggs, J., Dall'Ora, C., Schmidt, P. E., & Smith, G. B. (2019). Nurse staffing, nursing assistants and hospital mortality: Retrospective longitudinal cohort study. *BMJ Quality & Safety, 28*(8), 609–617. https://doi.org/10.1136/bmjqs-2018-008043

Kovner, C., Cheryl, J., Chunliu, Z., Peter, J. G., & Jayasree, B. (2002). Nurse staffing and postsurgical adverse events: An analysis of administrative data from a sample of U.S. hospitals, 1990–1996. *Health Services Research, 37*(3), 611–629. https://doi.org/10.1111/1475-6773.00040

Kovner, C., Mezey, M., & Harrington, C. (2000). Research priorities for staffing, case mix, and quality of care in U.S. nursing homes. *Journal of Nursing Scholarship, 32*(1), 77–80. https://doi.org/10.1111/j.1547-5069.2000.00077.x

Leclerc, L., Kennedy, K., & Campis, S. (2021). Human-centred leadership in health care: A contemporary nursing leadership theory generated via constructivist grounded theory. *Journal of Nursing Management, 29*(2), 294–306. doi:10.1111/jonm.13154

Leclerc, L., Kennedy, K., & Campis, S. (2022). *Human-centered leadership in health care: Evolution of a revolution.* Morgan James Publishing.

Lichtig, L. K., Knauf, R. A., & Milholland, D. K. (1999). Some impacts of nursing on acute care hospital outcomes. *Journal of Nursing Administration, 29*(2), 25–33. https://doi.org/10.1097/00005110-199902000-00008

Malloch, K., & Porter-O'Grady, T. (2019). *The leadership of nursing practice.* Jones & Bartlett Learning.

Mason, D. (2020). Nurses lack representation in media: recognize them for the leaders that they are. *USA Today.* https://www.usatoday.com/story/opinion/2020/06/26/nurses-leaders-medicine-but-overshadowed-media-column/3223242001/

Mason, D. J., Nixon, L., Glickstein, B., Han, S., Westphaln, K., & Carter, L. (2018). The Woodhull Study revisited: Nurses' representation in health news media 20 years later. *Journal of Nursing Scholarship, 50,* 695–704. https://doi.org/10.1111/jnu.12429

McHugh, M. D., Aiken, L. H., Sloane, D. M., Windsor, C., Douglas, C., & Yates, P. (2021). Effects of nurse-to-patient ratio legislation on nurse staffing and patient mortality, readmissions, and length of stay: A prospective study in a panel of hospitals. *The Lancet, 397*(10288), 1905–1913. https://doi.org/10.1016/S0140-6736(21)00768-6

Michel, A., Ryan, N., Mattheus, D., Branson, S., Hekel, B., & Fontenot, H. B. (2021). Undergraduate nursing students' perceptions on nursing education during the 2020 COVID-19 pandemic: A national sample. *Nursing Outlook, 69*(5), 903–912. https://doi.org/10.1016/j.outlook.2021.05.004

National Council of State Boards of Nursing. (n.d.). *Summary of modifications to the NCLEX-RN® and NCLEX-PN® examinations starting Oct. 1, 2020.* https://www.ncsbn.org/SummaryofModificationstoNCLEX.pdf

National Council of State Boards of Nursing. (2020). *Emergency declarations.* https://www.ncsbn.org/14582.htm#14521

Needleman, J., Buerhaus, P., Mattke, S., Stewart, M., & Zelevinsky, K. (2002). Nurse-staffing levels and the quality of care in hospitals. *New England Journal of Medicine, 346*(22), 1715–1722. https://doi.org/10.1056/NEJMsa012247

Needleman, J., Buerhaus, P., Pankratz, V. S., Leibson, C. L., Stevens, S. R., & Harris, M. (2011). Nurse staffing and inpatient hospital mortality. *New England Journal of Medicine, 364*(11), 1037–1045. https://doi.org/10.1056/NEJMsa1001025

Nundy, S. (2021). *Care after Covid: What the pandemic revealed is broken in healthcare and how to reinvent it.* McGraw Hill.

Pronovost, P. J., Jenckes, M. W., Dorman, T., Garrett, E., Breslow, M. J., Rosenfeld, B. A., Lipsett, P. A., & Bass, E. (1999). Organizational characteristics of intensive care units related to outcomes of abdominal aortic surgery. *JAMA, 281*(14), 1310–1317. https://doi.org/10.1001/jama.281.14.1310

Robbins, R., & Lesser, S. (2022). Abuse in the workplace. *Medscape Nurses*. https://www.medscape.com/slideshow/workplace-abuse-6014937

Saad, L. (2022). Military brass, judges among professions at new image lows. *Gallup Polls*. https://news.gallup.com/poll/388649/military-brass-judges-among-professions-new-image-lows.aspx

A
Stories of Leadership in Crisis

PROTOCOL TITLE: Stories of Leadership in Crisis

PRINCIPAL INVESTIGATOR:

Name: Carolyn Reilly
Department: School of Nursing

VERSION: Version 2 dated 8/26/20

FUNDING SOURCE: none

Table of Contents

1. Study Summary 3
2. Objectives 3
3. Background 3
4. Study Endpoints 3
5. Study Intervention / Design 3
6. Procedures Involved 4
7. Data and Specimen Banking 4
8. Sharing of Results with Participants 4
9. Study Timelines 5
10. Subject Population 5
11. Local Number of Participants 5
12. Recruitment Methods 6
13. Withdrawal of Participants 6
14. Risks to Participants 6
15. Potential Benefits to Participants 6
16. Data Analysis, Management and Confidentiality 6
17. Provisions to Monitor the Data to Ensure the Safety of Participants 7
18. Provisions to Protect the Privacy Interests of Participants and Confidentiality of Participants' identifiable data 7
19. Economic Burden to Participants 7
20. Consent Process 7
21. Setting 7
22. Resources Available 7
23. References ....

Stories of Leadership in Crisis

1. Study Summary

Study Title	Stories of Leadership in Crisis
Study Design	Qualitative
Primary Objective	To capture the crisis leadership stories of healthcare leaders using a crisis leadership framework
Secondary Objective(s)	
Research Intervention(s)/Interactions	Qualitative interviews only
Study Population	Nursing leaders from across Emory Healthcare and Mercy Care
Sample Size	10
Study Duration for individual participants	3 months
Study Specific Abbreviations/ Definitions	
Funding Source (if any)	none

2. Objectives

To capture the crisis leadership stories of healthcare leaders using a crisis leadership framework.

3. Background

Crisis is all the rage these days. As it should be. The United States and every member of the world community is experiencing an onrush of critical incidents and seminal change in a highly abbreviated time span (Blair, 2020). The problem with these events in this time of crisis is that it catches us by surprise, and the ordinary and usual practices and responses exercised in the management of ordinary change simply don't suffice. Crisis calls for extraordinary leadership compressed in a time frame that demands immediate action and exemplary leadership capacity. The problem is that most of us are not prepared either formally or experientially to quickly change our human dynamics and leader action to effectively and immediately respond to critical events as they emerge.

Leading in times of crisis like the recent pandemic, however, is a learned skill. The problem frequently is that it is not an often-utilized set of skills, so the skill set gets rusty the deeper it's embedded into the history of our leadership experience. Fortunately, the principles of leadership are constant and consistent. There are no new magic, emergent skills that are clothed in mystery and secrets that only the privileged can access, and this is just as true in the leadership of crisis (Northouse, 2018). However, the expression of leadership skills in a period of crisis has a different level of orientation and intensity that requires some drill-down and focus to be expressed appropriately and with impact.

In the March 4, 2020 issue of *Forbes* magazine, leadership contributor Davia Temin, drawing from critical leadership science (Diamond, 2019; Spector, 2019), pointed out the eight specific leadership capacities that serve us well in a crisis such as the pandemic of 2020 (Temin, 2020). Temin notes that this recent COVID pandemic disrupted every aspect of human life: social, political, business, professional, personal, and relational. Unlike the normal and ordinary course of events in our personal and work lives, brutally unusual circumstances like a pandemic catch us by surprise and bring the extraordinary into our lives creating mental, emotional, and physiologic distress. In a crisis, we feel out of control, unclear, multiply challenged, and unsure how to regain equilibrium (Cavaiola & Colford, 2017). It appears as though the rules change dramatically, and the ordinary tools we have for contending with the ongoing events of life no longer seem adequate to addressing new issues that we had not anticipated and that are currently beyond our scope of response. Of course, it helps considerably when long-term preparation has readied an organization for inevitable crisis with a well-designed structure for crisis response (Figure 1).

It is the onset of the crisis that creates this immediate disequilibrium. What does not happen is a sudden loss of capacity or potential viable response to the critical incidents we are confronting. It is the sense of being overwhelmed, immediately challenged, looking for different responses than would have normally emerged in the ordinary course of living one's life or doing one's work. The leadership skills essential to addressing the elements of a crisis and moving to appropriate response are the same as those expressed in any other leadership situation. In crisis they are merely heightened and intensified, and the timeline for their appropriate exercise is considerably shortened (Johnson, 2018). In addition, the number of leadership skill sets and variabilities diminish to a key few that ascend the leadership hierarchy and take prominence in their utility and viability for immediate problem-solving (Marcus et al., 2019).

The purpose of this project is to capture stories of healthcare leaders as they have managed during the Covid-19 pandemic. Questions have been developed to elicit stories based on the eight topical themes: managing denial, keeping head above water, creativity and innovation, teamwork, communication, information provided, leadership support, and grounding actions in evidence.

4. Study Endpoints

The study endpoints will be to gather five to six exemplars of crisis leadership from each leader. These vignettes should focus on both opportunities and challenges the mentor perceives from within their particular crisis situation. These will be developed into short chapters to be compiled into a book focused on leading in times of crisis.

5. Study Intervention/Design
   a. This study will involve qualitative interviews conducted by an Emory Nursing student and their assigned healthcare leader mentor. Students were previously paired with a leadership mentor in early 2020 prior to the Covid-19 pandemic. This pairing was outside of any research activities and is part of a Leadership Scholars Program at the Nell Hodgson Woodruff School of Nursing. Previously,

students were to work on a quality improvement project with their mentors. When the pandemic occurred, this new project was imagined as a way to preserve the integrity of a student honors project and to integrate aspects of crisis leadership into the program. Thus, students already have a relationship with the mentors who will be sharing their stories.

6. Procedures Involved
    a. Each student will conduct recorded, qualitative interviews with their leadership mentor (five to six sessions) for leadership issues that were experienced by the mentor during the crisis. These will be conducted via telephone or via Zoom.
    b. No long-term follow-up is anticipated. The leaders will be interviewed approximately six times.
    c. The students will use the questions developed as a class attached to this proposal. Interviews will be recorded and transcribed verbatim by the students. The recordings will not be preserved once transcribed. The transcriptions will not include any identifying information about the healthcare leader being interviewed.
    d. A thematic analysis will be done on all interviews by the students and the PI, producing vignettes to be used to illustrate crisis leadership theory.
    e. The vignettes will likely focus on both opportunities and challenges the mentor perceived from within their particular crisis situation. These will be developed into short chapters to be compiled into a book focused on leading in times of crisis. No leader participating in the interviews will be identified in the book, with only pseudonyms used.
    f. Participants will not be deceived in anyway and have already provided verbal consent to participate in the project. We will obtain written consent.

7. Data and Specimen Banking

No identifying data will be collected during the interviews. Interviews will be recorded and transcribed verbatim by the students. The recordings will not be preserved once transcribed. The transcriptions will not include any identifying information about the healthcare leader being interviewed. The recordings will be destroyed once transcription is complete by November 1, 2020. Transcripts will be stored on a secured, password-protected Emory Box site, with access only granted to study personnel and students (also approved by IRB).

8. Sharing of Results With Participants

Results will only be shared with participants once the book has been published. Participants will be given a copy of the book.

9. Study Timelines

The subjects will be interviewed five to six times for their stories using the questions attached. These interviews should be approximately one hour in length each. The subjects (healthcare leaders) already have a relationship with the students and meet with them presently in their capacity as leadership mentors.

10. Subject Population
Inclusion criteria: previously assigned leadership mentors working at Emory Healthcare, CDC, and Mercy Care

Exclusion criteria: NA

11. Local Number of Participants
10

12. Recruitment Methods
As previously described, there is no recruitment. Ten Emory nursing students are enrolled as leadership scholars. They have previously been assigned mentors (from Emory Healthcare, Mercy Care, the CDC, and Emory University) who agreed to mentor them through their senior year with a leadership project. These mentors have all agreed with this combined project to share their stories of leadership in crisis with the students and have them recorded.

13. Withdrawal of Participants
It is not anticipated that any mentor will be withdrawn from their role as a leadership mentor. Their stories may not be included in the final version of the book.

Should a mentor decide that they do not want a portion of their interview transcribed for inclusion in the analysis and book, we will honor this request.

14. Risks to Participants
The only foreseeable risks include 1) possible emotional stress from discussing a crisis situation; and 2) inadvertent risks of loss of privacy or breach of confidentiality.

For emotional stress, the leader will be referred to the Faculty and Staff Assistance Program.

To prevent loss of privacy or breach of confidentiality, recordings will be anonymously collected without stating name, date, or location and only kept by the student until transcribed. No identifying information will be transcribed and only pseudonyms used. Transcripts will be stored on a secured, password-protected Emory Box site with access only granted to study personnel and students (also approved by IRB).

15. Potential Benefits to Participants
No direct benefit is anticipated, though the healthcare leader may receive some benefit from recounting events and reexamining them.

No compensation will be provided to any participant.

16. Data Analysis, Management, and Confidentiality

Qualitative thematic analysis of the transcripts will be undertaken. Transcripts will be stored through study completion and a book published in accordance with IRB rules.

17. Provisions to Monitor the Data to Ensure the Safety of Participants

NA – no more than minimal risk

18. <u>Provisions to Protect the Privacy Interests of Participants and Confidentiality of Participants' identifiable Data</u>

No identifiable data will be collected. The students will record the interviews on their phones and delete them upon transcription of the interview. No identifying information will be included in the written transcript. These will be stored on a secured, password-protected Emory Box site with access only granted to study personnel and students (also approved by IRB).

19. Economic Burden to Participants

No costs are anticipated.

20. Consent Process

Participant consent will be obtained verbally using the approved IRB verbal consent.

21. Setting

Interview will take place via Zoom or telephone at a time convenient to the mentor and student.

22. Resources Available

This project is part of a leadership class in which the concepts of crisis leadership are being taught, along with principles related to qualitative interviewing and thematic analysis. The students are completing citi training to assure human subject protection. The course is a one-hour credit course, and students are expected to devote approximately 30 hours over the course of the semester to this project. Mentor time commitment is approximately five hours a month from March–December; however, only a small percentage of that time is devoted to this project. Mentors will spend about six hours being interviewed over the span of three months.

23. References

Blair, S. (2020). *10 years to midnight: For urgent global crises in their strategic solutions*. Barrett Koehler.

Cavaiola, A., & Colford, J. (2017). *Crisis intervention: A practical guide*: Sage Publications.

Diamond, J. (2019). *Crisis*. Penguin Random House.

Johnson, T. J. (2018). *Crisis leadership: How to lead in times of crisis, threat and uncertainty*. Bloomsbury Business.

Marcus, L., McNulty, E., Henderson, J., Dorn, B., & Gergen, D. (2019). *Your it: Crisis, change, and how to lead when it matters most*. Perseus Books.

Northouse, P. (2018). *Leadership: Theory and practice* (8th ed.). Sage Publications.

Spector, B. (2019). *Constructing crisis: Leaders, crises, and claims of urgency*. Cambridge University Press.

Temin, D. (2020). Crisis leadership in real time: 8 pandemic best practices. *Forbes*. https://www.forbes.com/sites/daviatemin/2020/03/04/crisis-leadership-in-real-time-8-pandemic-best-practices/#72fbfc59797e

B
Oral Consent Script for a Research Study

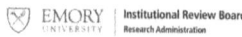

Emory University
Oral Consent Script
For a Research Study

<u>Study Title</u>:   Stories of Leadership in Crisis
<u>IRB #</u>: 00001360
<u>Principal Investigator</u>:   Carolyn Miller Reilly, PhD, RN, CHFN-K, CNE, FAHA, FAAN

<u>Introduction and Study Overview</u>

Thank you for your interest in our qualitative research study. We would like to tell you everything you need to think about before you decide whether or not to join the study. It is entirely your choice. If you decide to take part, you can change your mind later on and withdraw from the research study.

The purpose of this study is to capture the crisis leadership stories of healthcare leaders using a crisis leadership framework. This study will take about five to six hours to complete.

If you join, you will be asked to participate in five to six interviews by your leadership student mentee concerning healthcare leadership situations during the Covid-19 crisis. The student will ask you specific questions and then record your answers. At no time will you be identified during the recording, and you do not need to disclose any identifying information such as the specific group you work with or the hospital. The recordings will be transcribed by the student, and a pseudonym will be used if necessary for your own name and healthcare facility and unit.

The transcripts from all interviews will be evaluated for themes and stories gathered to describe components of crisis leadership. A crisis leadership textbook will be developed, and your stories may be a part of this textbook.

<u>Possible risks include</u>:
1)   Possible emotional stress from discussing a crisis situation. Should this occur, we will refer you to the Faculty and Staff Assistance Program at Emory University.
2)   Inadvertent risks of loss of privacy or breach of confidentiality. To prevent loss of privacy or breach of confidentiality, recordings will be anonymously collected without stating name, date, or location and only kept by the student until transcribed. No identifying information will be transcribed and only pseudonyms used. Transcripts will be stored on a secured, password-protected Emory Box site with access only granted to study personnel and students.

<u>Benefits include</u>:
This study is not designed to benefit you directly. This study is designed to learn more about healthcare crisis leadership. The study results may be used to help others in the future.

<u>Compensation</u>:
You will not be offered payment for being in this study.

B → Oral Consent Script for a Research Study

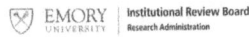

Other options outside this study:
You do not have to be in this study to be a leadership scholar mentor.

Confidentiality:
Certain offices and people other than the researchers may look at study records. Government agencies and Emory employees overseeing proper study conduct may look at your study records. These offices include the Office for Human Research Protections, the funder(s), the Emory Institutional Review Board, and the Emory Office of Compliance. Emory will keep any research records we create private to the extent we are required to do so by law. A study number rather than your name will be used on study records wherever possible. Your name and other facts that might point to you will not appear when we present this study or publish its results.

Study records can be opened by court order. They may also be produced in response to a subpoena or a request for production of documents.

Storing and sharing your information:
De-identified data from this study (data that has been stripped of all information that can identify you) may be placed into public databases where, in addition to having no direct identifiers, researchers will need to sign data use agreements before accessing the data. We will remove or code any personal information that could identify you before your information is shared. This will ensure that, by current scientific standards and known methods, it is extremely unlikely that anyone would be able to identify you from the information we share. Despite these measures, we cannot guarantee anonymity of your personal data.

Your data from this study will not be shared with anyone outside this study, even if we take out all the information that can identify you.

We will use your sample and data only for research. We will not sell them. However, the results of this research might someday lead to the development of products (such as a textbook) that could be sold by a company. You will not receive money from the sale of any such product.

Once the study has been completed, we will send you a summary of all of the results of the study and what they mean. We will not send you your individual results from this study.

Underline: Withdrawal from the study:
You have the right to leave a study at any time without penalty.

Underline: Contact information
Contact Dr. Carolyn Reilly at xxx-xxx-xxxx:
- If you have any questions about this study or your part in it
- If you have questions or concerns about the research

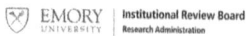

Contact the Emory Institutional Review Board at 404-712-0720 or 877-503-9797 or irb@emory.edu:
- If you have questions about your rights as a research participant
- If you have complaints about the research or an issue you rather discuss with someone outside the research team

You may also let the IRB know about your experience as a research participant through our Research Participant Survey at https://tinyurl.com/ycewgkke.

Consent and authorization
Consent

Do you have any questions about anything I just said? Were there any parts that seemed unclear?

Do you agree to take part in the study?

Participant agrees to participate: Yes   No

If Yes:

_____
Name of participant

_____   _____ _____
Signature of person conducting informed consent discussion   Date   Time

_____
Name of person conducting informed consent discussion

C
Questions for Mentor Interviews Regarding Crisis Leadership

TOPICAL THEMES

1. Managing denial:

    - When did you first know this was going to be a crisis?

    - What are you/your unit/your hospital doing to support your staff holistically during the Covid-19 crisis?

2. Keeping head above water; staying in control. Emotional intelligence:

    - How did you feel about being overwhelmed?

3. Creativity and innovation:

    - What were some initial changes you had to make as a leader in order to respond to the emerging situation Covid-19 was presenting?

    - When you were flying by the seat of your pants, can you identify one thing you did to deal with the crisis?

    - What kinds of gaps in planning became apparent as a result of responding to Covid-19? In other words, what situations or challenges emerged that had been overlooked when planning for a crisis?

4. Team (people who can be depended on):

    - Who did you trust to work with during this crisis?

5. Communication (the "how"—the methodology):

    - What strategies did you use to inform staff of changes that were occurring to prevent confusion or resistance to change?

    - What was unique about the communication of information during Covid-19 that is different from normal circumstances?

C → Questions for Mentor Interviews Regarding Crisis Leadership

6. Information provided (the "what"—the structural elements):
   - What information did you rely on to help guide your actions as a leader responding to Covid-19?
   - Who/what were your trusted information sources, and how did they guide your planning and response?
   - Did the information change, and how did you deal with the change? (example: complete reversal on public wearing masks)

7. Leaders are crisis leaders but are not alone in the crisis—is this really interdepartmental agency and connectivity?
   - Who supported you in the organization?
   - What partnerships did you develop among other groups within the organization?
   - What other departments have you been working closely with, and how have these relationships changed through the crisis?
   - What were unexpected collaborations and partnerships that developed?

8. Grounding actions in evidence:
   - What sources/data/information did you use to determine changes in policies and procedures?
     - Were these evidenced-based?
       - Examples of those that were and those that were not
       - Anecdotal examples
   - How did things change as new guidelines developed?
   - How did you handle new revelations or guidelines about treating the virus?

CHRONOLOGICAL/SEQUENTIAL (BEGINNING, MIDDLE, AND END)

Interested in their perception—their insight, sense, feeling. Good to start with:

> How do you feel about what has happened?

Background—getting to know mentor:

1. What was your primary role before Covid-19?
2. What was your primary role through the Covid-19 crisis?
3. Did your role shift at all?
4. What is your definition of being a leader?
5. How does your role intertwine with other leadership roles?
6. What training or protocol did your organization have in place for managing an epidemic or pandemic prior to Covid-19? When did you know about the organizational plan for emergency response prior to Covid?

Covid initial phase (retrospective):

1. When did you first know this was going to be a crisis?
2. How was this communicated to you?

Covid plateau phase (currently in this phase)—perhaps even resurgence:

1. Did your role change? Did your style change during this crisis?
2. How do you feel about the current unforeseen daily challenges?
3. How has your leadership changed/ shifted during this crisis?

Covid anticipated recovery phase/planning for future:

1. How would you better prepared in the future?
2. What have you learned from this experience that would inform your future crisis leadership?

Index

A

accountability, 187–188, 221
accuracy, 141–144
achievement, 58
action, promoting, 149–150
active listening, 72
adaptability, 75–76
    adaptive leadership, 76–89 (*see also* adaptive leadership)
    high reliability organizations (HROs), 217–220
    preparation to adaptation, 205–217
    skills, 57, 58 (*see also* self-management)
adaptive challenges, 95–96
adaptive coping, 240, 246
adaptive leadership, 76–89
    being present, 90
    building on the past, 77, 78–80
    conveying strategic intent, 93–94
    decision-making, 91–92
    experimentation, 77, 80–83
    focusing on missions, 92–93
    persistence, 77, 87–89
    relying on diversity, 77, 83–85
    remodeling, 89–94
    re-regulating, 77, 85–87
adaptive models, 205
adaptive phase, 213–217
advocacy, 35, 36
affiliation, 35, 36
Agbanyim, J. Ibeh, 169
Agbanyim's principles of collaboration, 169
Agency for Healthcare Research and Quality (AHRQ), 168
American Association of Colleges of Nursing (AACN), 24
American Association of Critical-Care Nurses (AACN), 129
American College of Healthcare Executives, 25

American Nurses Association (ANA), 25, 231
American Nurses Foundation New Pulse, 27
American Organization for Nursing Leadership (AONL), 265, 266
American Psychological Association (APA), 52, 232
appearance, 35, 36
application
  of emotional intelligence (EI), 51–52
  of leadership styles, 119–121, 122
areas of improvement, 20, 97–98, 226
asking for help, 13–14
assessing
  emotional intelligence (EI), 72
  institutional support, 132
  mentor relationships, 46
  self-management, 71
association, 35, 36
attack on Pearl Harbor, 137, 138–139
authentic leadership, 32
authoritative/visionary leadership style, 110
autocratic leadership style, 109
Awakener (leadership), 268

B

balancing effective care, 81
Beghetto, Robert, 102, 103, 104
behavior. *See also* skills
  Hackman, J. Richard, 168
  leadership characteristics, 3–4, 109
  new patterns of, 77
Behavioral Theories of Leadership, 107
being present, 90
Beldoch, Michael, 52
bi-directional communication, 147. *See also* communication
Black nurses, 27. *See also* diversity
BP oil spill (2010), 137
Brown, Brené, 66
building on the past, 77, 78–80

C

capacities
  applying evidence/emotional intelligence, 14–16
  asking for help, 13–14
  communication, 9–11
  conveying critical information, 12–13
  innovation, 7–8
  of leadership, 4–17
  managing denial, 5–6
  role and expectation setting, 8–9
  self-awareness, 58
  triaging priorities, 6–7
Care After Covid: What the Pandemic Revealed Is Broken in Healthcare and How to Reinvent It (Nundy), 271
Centers for Disease Control and Prevention (CDC), 78, 83, 103, 139, 140, 149, 195, 206, 261
change
  adaptive leadership and, 76 (*see also* adaptive leadership)
  areas of improvement, 226
  continuity, 193–194 (*see also* continuity)
  correcting course, 224–225
  discomfort of change, 225
  focusing on positive, 188
  high reliability organizations (HROs), 226
  integrating, 201–203
  Lewin's Change Model Theory, 199–200
  Maurer's Levels of Resistance and Change Model, 198, 200
  Nudge Theory, 199, 200
  opportunity to change roles, 263–264
  positive, 237, 240
  standardization, 193–194 (*see also* standardization)
  success, 221
  theory due to rapid modification, 198–200

characteristics of leadership, 3–4
checklists, coping, 241
chief nursing officers, chief nursing executives (CNOs/CNEs), 266
clinical nurses, 188–189. *See also* leadership; nursing
coaching, Hackman's Team Coaching Model, 168–169. *See also* mentoring
Cochrane Systematic Reviews, 142
code-switching, 33–35, 45
collaboration, 163–164. *See also* teamwork
    Agbanyim's principles of collaboration, 169
    Agency for Healthcare Research and Quality (AHRQ), 168
    clarifying concepts, 164–165
    commitments to diversity, 179–183
    commitments to shared mission, 171–174
    communication, 177–178
    definition of, 164
    effective, 189
    Hackman's Team Coaching Model, 168–169
    Incident Command System (ICS), 165–167, 190
    mentoring, 183–186
    models, 170
    motivation, 183–186, 190
    positive leadership, 183–186
    principles for, 167–169
    roles and responsibilities, 178–179
    trust and, 174–176
commitments
    to diversity, 179–183
    to resilience, 219
    to shared missions, 171–174
communication
    asking for help, 13–14
    collaboration, 177–178
    conveying critical information, 12–13
    conveying strategic intent, 93–94
    during crises, 136–139
    definition of, 136
    encouraging open, 187
    errors, 160
    leadership skills, 9–11
    modes of, 155–158
    multifaceted, 135–136 (*see also* multifaceted communication)
    personal communication challenges, 19
    planning, 160
    principles of crisis communication, 139–153
    reassurance, 153–154
    self-assessments, 159–160
    skills, 3–4
    transparency, 153–154, 221
    Zoom, 63
Community Resiliency Model (CRM), 250, 251
Complex Adaptive Systems Model, 203
components of nursing leadership, 187–189
    connecting to roles, 188–189
    emphasizing accountability, 187–188
    encouraging open communication, 187
    focusing on positive change, 188
    supporting continued learning, 187
concepts, clarifying, 164–165
confidence, 103
connectedness, mission of, 115, 247
Connector (leadership), 268–269
Contingency Theory of Leadership, 107
continued learning, supporting, 187
continuity, 193–194
    change theory due to rapid modification, 198–200
    high reliability organizations (HROs), 217–220
    integrating change, 201–203
    Lewin's Change Model Theory, 199–200
    Maurer's Levels of Resistance and Change Model, 198, 200
    Nudge Theory, 199, 200
    organizational, 195–197
    organizational stability, 220–222
    preparation to adaptation, 205–217
coordination, Incident Command System (ICS), 165–167
coping, 231–232

adaptive, 240, 246
checklists, 241
positive change, 237
roles, 240
trauma, 236–237
coronavirus, 207. *See also* Covid-19 pandemic
covering, 35–36, 42
Covid-19 pandemic, 1, 29, 51, 61, 62, 63, 64, 65, 80, 92, 93, 120, 152, 231, 261
creativity in, 101 (*see also* creativity)
crisis communication, 140
innovation in the Covid era, 129–130
integrating change during, 201–203
responses to, 207
creative action framework, 104
creative leadership, 105–112
leadership theory and, 105–112
styles, 106–111
THNK School of Creative Leadership, 112
creativity
constructs that foster, 113
in crises, 101–104
definition of, 102
fostering, 122–129
innovation in the Covid era, 129–130
leadership styles and, 119–121, 122
mutual trust, 117–118, 122
risk, 103
self-assessments, 131
shared commitments, 114–116, 122
solid foundation of, 113–121
supporting others, 132–133
credibility, 144–146
crises
areas of improvement, 226
attack on Pearl Harbor, 137, 138–139
BP oil spill (2010), 137
communication during, 136–139
correcting course, 224–225
Covid-19 pandemic, 231 (*see* Covid-19 pandemic)
creative leadership in (*see* creative leadership)
creativity in, 101–104 (*see also* creativity)
discomfort of change, 225
fostering creativity, 122–129
fostering innovation, 122–129
foundation for creativity in, 113–121
high reliability organizations (HROs), 226
Incident Command System (ICS), 165–167
innovation in, 101–104 (*see also* innovation)
integrating change, 201–203
Johnson & Johnson's (J&J) product tampering (1982), 137
leadership, 103 (*see also* crisis leadership; leadership)
models, 205–217
nursing shortages, 265–266
organizational continuity, 195–197
principles of crisis communication, 139–153
responses to, 1, 2
stories of leadership in crisis, 277–284
timelines for, 211
Crisis and Emergency Risk Communication (CERC) manual, 139, 140
crisis leadership, 103
applying evidence/emotional intelligence, 14–16
asking for help, 13–14
capacities, 4–17
communication, 9–11
conveying critical information, 12–13
innovation, 7–8
leadership characteristics, 3–4
managing denial, 5–6
principles of, 1
responses to crises, 2
role and expectation setting, 8–9
structural tools, 17
triaging priorities, 6–7
critical information, conveying, 12–13
cultural intelligence (CQ), 40–41
cultural racism, definition of, 26

D

death, pandemics and, 231, 232
decision-making, 3, 75–76, 210
   adaptive leadership, 91–92
   innovations, 117–118
deference to expertise, 220
deliberate reflection, 237–248, 252–253
democratic/transformational leadership style, 111
demographics, race, 24
denial, managing, 5–6
development
   cultural intelligence (CQ), 40–41
   of emotional intelligence (EI), 51–52 (*see also* emotional intelligence [EI])
   leadership skill strategies, 36–39
disasters, 195. *See also* crises
disciplinarity concepts, 180–181
discrimination, 24. *See also* racism
   addressing, 25
   definition of, 26
diversity, 23–24
   addressing racism, 25–27
   authentic leadership, 32
   commitments to, 179–183
   cultural intelligence (CQ), 40–41
   healthcare inequity and, 24–25
   historically marginalized groups (HMGs), 33–36
   leadership skill development strategies, 36–39
   mentor experience with race, 28–31
   power and racism, 27–28
   relying on, 77, 83–85
diversity, equity, and inclusion (DEI), 24, 27, 29, 44
domains, posttraumatic growth (PTG), 234–235, 238–239
Dunning, Christine, 247

E

Ebola, 79, 80
economic instability, 231
effective communication, 151, 159–160. *See also* communication
emergency models, 205
emergency phase, 210–213
emotional intelligence (EI), 14–16, 241
   assessing, 72
   definition of, 52
   development of, 51–52
   Goleman's Model of, 53–69 (*see also* Goleman's Model of EI)
   in nursing, 69
Emotional Intelligence: Why It Can Matter More Than IQ (Goleman), 53
The Emotionally Intelligent Leader (Goleman), 53
emotional self-control, 58
empathy, 66–68, 146–148
encouraging open communication, 187
engagement, 3
Environment of Care section (Joint Commission), 78
errors, communication, 160
ethnicity, 23, 35. *See also* diversity
evaluating strategies, 97
evidence, applying, 14–16
examples, priorities, 18
expectation setting, 8–9
experimentation, 77, 80–83
expertise
   deference to, 220
   valuing, 117–118
external coping, 236–237

F

failure, preoccupation with, 218
fear, 231

Federal Emergency Management Agency (FEMA), 165, 166
Federal Highway Administration, 165
Federally Qualified Health Centers, 152
focus groups, 267
focusing on missions, 92–93
Forbes magazine, 4
frameworks
  Beghetto's creative action, 104
  for emotional intelligence (EI), 52
Future of Nursing 2020–2030 report, 25

G

gender identity, 24, 28, 35
geographic residence, 24
George Washington University, 273
Georgia Department of Public Health, 210
goals, breaking down, 71
Goffman, Erving, 33
Goleman, Daniel J., 53–69. *See also* Goleman's Model of EI
Goleman's Model of EI, 53–69
  empathy (social-awareness and), 66–68
  motivation, 64–65
  self-awareness, 53–57
  self-management, 57–64
governance, nursing, 270–271
Great Man Theory of Leadership, 106, 109
groups
  collaboration, 164 (*see also* collaboration)
  focus, 267
growth, 231–232. *See also* posttraumatic growth (PTG) theory

H

Hackman, J. Richard, 168
Hackman's Team Coaching Model, 168–169
healthcare inequity, 24–25. *See also* diversity
heart, leading from, 32. *See also* leadership
Heifetz Model, 78
help, asking for, 13–14
hidden power concept, 28
hierarchies, 219. *See also* managing
high reliability organizations (HROs), 217–220, 226
  commitment to resilience, 219
  deference to expertise, 220
  preoccupation with failure, 218
  reluctance to simplify, 218–219
  sensitivity to operations, 219
Hispanic/Latino nurses, 27. *See also* diversity
historically marginalized groups (HMGs), 33–36
How to Win Friends & Influence People (Carnegie), 185–186
Human-Centered Leadership, 267, 269
Human-Centered Leadership in Healthcare: Evolution of a Revolution (Watson), 267

I

identifying mentor relationships, 46
Implicit Association Test (IAT), 45
improvement
  areas of, 20, 97–98
  motivation, 65
  performance, 58, 263
  self-awareness, 57
  self-management, 64
  social awareness, 68
Incident Command System (ICS), 165–167, 190, 195, 203, 261, 267
inclusion, 179–183

inequity
  healthcare, 24–25 (*see also* diversity)
  racial, 28 (*see also* race)
influenza, 195, 196
initiative, taking, 58
innovation, 7–8, 77, 179
  in the Covid era, 129–130
  decision-making, 117–118
  definition of, 102
  fostering, 122–129
  planning, 210
  self-assessments, 131
  supporting others, 132–133
instinct, trusting, 70
institutional support, assessing, 132
integrating change, 201–203
interdisciplinary concept, 180
internal coping, 236–237
International Council of Nurses (ICN), 231, 232
interviews, questions for (mentoring), 289–292
intradisciplinary concept, 180
invisible power concept, 28
isolation, 231

J–K

Johnson & Johnson's (J&J), 137
Joint Commission, 78, 165
Joint Commission on Accreditation of Healthcare Organizations (JCAHO), 195

Kemp, Brian P., 210
knowledge, 40, 179–183
knowns/unknowns, 91, 92

L

laissez-faire leadership style, 110
leadership
  adaptive, 76–89 (*see also* adaptive leadership)
  addressing racism, 25–27
  applying evidence/emotional intelligence, 14–16
  asking for help, 13–14
  authentic, 32
  Awakener, 268
  Behavioral Theories of Leadership, 107
  behavior characteristics, 109
  capacities, 4–17
  characteristics, 3–4
  communication, 9–11, 136–139 (*see also* communication)
  components of nursing, 187–189
  Connector, 268–269
  Contingency Theory of Leadership, 107
  conveying critical information, 12–13
  creative (*see* creative leadership)
  crises, 103
  cultural intelligence (CQ), 40–41
  diversity, 23–24 (*see also* diversity)
  empathy, 66–68
  expectation setting, 8–9
  governance structures, 270–271
  Great Man Theory of Leadership, 106, 109
  historically marginalized groups (HMGs), 33–39
  Human-Centered Leadership Model, 267, 269
  Incident Command System (ICS), 165–167, 190
  innovation, 7–8
  managing denial, 5–6
  mentor experience with race, 28–31
  motivation, 64–65
  nursing, 266–270
  planning, 210
  positive, 183–186
  posttraumatic growth (PTG) theory, 241, 248–251
  power and racism, 27–28
  principles of crisis, 1
  qualities, 1
  responses to crises, 2
  roles, 8–9, 166

self-awareness, 53–57
self-management, 57–64
skill development strategies, 36–39
social-awareness, 66–68
stories of leadership in crisis, 277–284
structural tools, 17
styles, 109–111, 117, 119–121, 122, 131
theories, 105–112
Trait Theory of Leadership, 106
Transactional Theory of Leadership, 108
Transformational Theory of Leadership, 108
triaging priorities, 6–7
Upholder, 269–270
working with teams, 186
lessons learned, 259–262
Leuner, B., 52
Lewin, Kurt, 199
Lewin's Change Model Theory, 199–200
licensure, 272

M

managing
    denial, 5–6
    management hierarchies, 165 (see also teamwork)
    self-management, 57–64
mapping (mentorship), 38
mask policies, 210. See also pandemics
Maslow's Hierarchy for provision of safety, 79
Maurer's Levels of Resistance and Change Model, 198, 200
Medicare, 165
mental and physical resets, 262
mental models, 247
mentoring. See also leadership
    collaboration, 183–186
    experience with race, 28–31
    importance of, 36–37
    mutual exchange model of reciprocal mentoring, 37
    practices, 37–39
    questions for interviews, 289–292
    relationships, 46
military leaders, 89
mindfulness, 246
minorities, 23, 33–36. See also diversity; historically marginalized groups (HMGs)
missions
    commitments to shared missions, 171–174
    connectedness, 115, 247
    focusing on, 92–93
    shared commitments, 114–116, 122
models. See also theories
    adaptive, 205
    collaboration, 170
    Community Resiliency Model (CRM), 250, 251
    Complex Adaptive Systems, 203
    crises, 205–217
    emergency, 205
    Goleman's Model of EI, 53–69 (see also Goleman's Model of EI)
    Hackman's Team Coaching, 168–169
    Heifetz, 78
    Human-Centered Leadership, 269
    leadership, 266–270
    Lewin's Change Model Theory, 199–200
    Maurer's Levels of Resistance and Change Model, 198, 200
    mental, 247
    Nudge Theory, 199, 200
    preparation, 205
    Revised Model of Posttraumatic Growth, 239
    skill set role, 19
modes of communication, 155–158. See also communication
motivation, 40
    collaboration, 183–186, 190
    Goleman's Model of EI, 64–65
    teamwork, 190
multidisciplinary concept, 180

multifaceted communication, 135–136
  during crises, 136–139
  modes of, 155–158
  principles of crisis communication, 139–153
  reassurance, 153–154
  transparency, 153–154
mutual exchange model of reciprocal mentoring, 37
mutual trust, 117–118, 122

N

National Academy of Medicine (NAM), 24
National Commission to Address Racism in Nursing, 26
National Council of State Boards of Nursing (NCSBN), 272
National Incident Management System (NIMS), 165, 195
Nation's Nurses Survey, 27
NextGen examination, 272
Nietzsche, Friedrich, 237
NIMs training, 261
Nudge Theory, 199, 200
Nundy, Shantanu, 271
Nurse Licensure Compact (NLC), 272
nurses of color (NOC), 25, 26
nursing. *See also* leadership
  components of leadership, 187–189
  emotional intelligence (EI) in, 69
  leadership, 266–270
  organizational stability, 220–222
  professional governance structures, 270–271
  shortages, 265–266

O

Obama, Barack, 78, 147
operations, sensitivity to, 219
opportunity to change roles, 263–264

optimism, 58, 62, 63
oral consent scripts, 285–288
organizational continuity, 195–197
organizational stability, 220–222
organizations, posttraumatic growth (PTG) theory in, 248–251
outcomes, 179, 232—237
ownership, 221

P

pacesetter leadership style, 111
pandemics, 51, 62, 196. *See also* Covid-19 pandemic; crises
  integrating change, 201–203
  need for social-awareness during, 66
  planning, 196–197
Parks, Sharon Daloz, 77
PDCA (Plan, Do, Check, and Act), 193, 194
people of color (POC), 27, 28
performance, improvement, 58, 263
persistence, adaptive leadership, 77, 87–89
personal communication challenges, 19
persons of influence (PI), 43–45
perspectives, commitments to diverse, 179–183
phases
  adaptive, 213–217
  of creative leadership, 112
  emergency, 210–213
  preparation, 206–210
planning
  communication, 160
  innovation, 210
  leadership, 210
  pandemics, 196–197
  response, 216
policies, revising, 214
positive change, 237, 240
positive leadership, 183–186
positive outcomes to trauma, 240
post-pandemic, 273. *See also* pandemics
posttraumatic growth (PTG) theory, 231–232, 234–235, 253–254

adaptive coping, 240
deliberate reflection, 237–248
domains, 238–239
leadership, 241
in organizations, 248–251
social support, 242–248
teamwork, 242
posttraumatic stress disorder (PTSD), 233
power
over concept, 28
and racism, 27–28
preoccupation with failure, 218
preparation
to adaptation, 205–217
models, 205
phases, 206–210
present, being, 90
principles for collaboration, 167–169
Agbanyim's principles of collaboration, 169
Agency for Healthcare Research and Quality (AHRQ), 168
Hackman's Team Coaching Model, 168–169
principles of crisis communication, 139–153
be credible, 144–146
be first, 140–141
be right, 141–144
express empathy, 146–148
promote action, 149–150
show respect, 151–153
principles of crisis leadership, 1
capacities, 4–17
leadership characteristics, 3–4
responses to crises, 2
priorities
examples, 18
pyramids, 18
triaging, 6–7
procedures, establishing, 247
profound uncertainty, creativity in, 102. *See also* creativity
protection (mentorship), 39
Public Health Emergency of International Concern, 207
pyramids, priorities, 18

Q–R

qualities
of coping checklist, 241
leadership, 1
questions for interviews (mentoring), 289–292

race, 23. *See also* diversity
authentic leadership, 32
awareness of, 42–43
code-switching, 33–35
covering, 35–36
definition of, 26
demographics, 24
disparities, 25
historically marginalized groups (HMGs), 33–36
mentor experience with, 28–31
racism
addressing, 24, 25–27
definition of, 26
power and, 27–28
rapid change, 193–194. *See also* change; crises
areas of improvement, 226
change theory due to, 198–200
correcting course, 224–225
discomfort of change, 225
high reliability organizations (HROs), 226
Lewin's Change Model Theory, 199–200
Maurer's Levels of Resistance and Change Model, 198, 200
Nudge Theory, 199, 200
reaching out, 46
Reagan, Ronald, 83, 183
reassurance, 153–154
re-evaluation, 263
reflection
deliberate, 237–248, 252–253
and re-evaluation, 263
relationships, 106
focused leadership style, 110
mentoring, 46
relaxation, 246

religious affiliations, 35
reluctance to simplify, 218–219
relying on diversity, 77, 83–85
remodeling adaptive leadership, 89–94
    being present, 90
    conveying strategic intent, 93–94
    decision-making, 91–92
    focusing on missions, 92–93
re-regulating, adaptive leadership, 77, 85–87
research, 267
    oral consent scripts, 285–288
resets, mental and physical, 262
resilience, 216, 231–232, 254
    commitments to, 219
    Community Resiliency Model (CRM), 250, 251
    teamwork, 242
    trauma, 233
respect, showing, 151–153
responses
    to crises, 1, 2
    planning, 216
responsibilities, collaboration, 178–179
Revised Model of Posttraumatic Growth, 239
revising policies, 214
risk, 103, 179
roles
    collaboration, 178–179
    connecting to, 188–189
    coping, 240
    hierarchies of, 166
    Incident Command System (ICS), 165–167, 190
    leadership, 8–9, 166
    opportunity to change, 263–264
    setting, 8–9
    skill set role models, 19
Roosevelt, Franklin D., 137, 138–139
rules, establishing, 247

S

self-assessments. *See also* assessing
    communication, 159–160
    creativity, 131
    innovation, 131
    leadership styles, 131
self-awareness, 53–57, 106
self-discipline, 32
self-inquiry, 106
self-management, 57–64, 71
self-regulation, 57, 62. *See also* self-management
sensitivity to operations, 219
sexual orientation, 24, 28, 35
shared missions, commitments to, 171–174. *See also* missions
shared visions, 106, 114–116
Sherman, Rose, 89
simplifying, reluctance to, 218–219
skills
    active listening, 72
    adaptability, 57, 58 (*see also* self-management)
    applying evidence/emotional intelligence, 14–16
    asking for help, 13–14
    communication, 3–4, 9–11
    conveying critical information, 12–13
    crisis leadership, 4–17
    goals (*see* goals)
    innovation, 7–8
    leadership, 3–4 (*see also* leadership)
    leadership skill development strategies, 36–39
    managing denial, 5–6
    role and expectation setting, 8–9
    triaging priorities, 6–7
skill set role models, 19
Skype, 158. *See also* Zoom
SMART (Specific, Measurable, Achievable, Realistic, and Time-Bound), 38, 46
social-awareness, empathy and, 66–68
social skills, 66
social support, 242–248

socioeconomic status, 35
stability, organizational, 220–222
staffing shortages, 265–266
standardization, 193–194
    high reliability organizations (HROs), 217–220
    need for, 203–205
    organizational stability, 220–222
    preparation to adaptation, 205–217
STARR technique, 20, 97–98, 190
STOP technique, 246
stories, 247
    of leadership in crisis, 277–284
strategic intent, conveying, 93–94
strategies
    concept of, 40
    evaluating, 97
    leadership skill development, 36–39
    positive change, 237
stress, relief of, 246
structural racism, definition of, 26
structural tools, crisis leadership, 17
styles of leadership, 109–111, 117, 119–121, 122, 131
success, change, 221
Sunstein, Cass, 199
support
    continued learning, 187
    others (creativity/innovation), 132–133
    posttraumatic growth (PTG) theory, 242–248
    the transition (mentorship), 39

T

taking initiative, 58
teaching the job (mentorship), 39
teamwork, 163–164
    clarifying concepts, 164–165
    components of nursing leadership, 187–189
    definition of, 164
    effective, 189
    Hackman's Team Coaching Model, 168–169
    Incident Command System (ICS), 165–167, 190
    involvement, 3
    motivation, 190
    posttraumatic growth (PTG) theory, 242
    resiliency, 242
    working with teams, 186
technical challenges, 95–96
Technical Resources, Assistance Center, and Information Exchange (TRACIE), 261, 263
Temin, Davia, 4
Thaler, Richard, 199
theories
    Behavioral Theories of Leadership, 107
    Contingency Theory of Leadership, 107
    Great Man Theory of Leadership, 106, 109
    leadership, 105–112
    Nudge Theory, 199, 200
    posttraumatic growth (PTG), 231–232, 234–235, 237–248 (see also posttraumatic growth (PTG) theory)
    Trait Theory of Leadership, 106
    Transactional Theory of Leadership, 108
    Transformational Theory of Leadership, 108
THNK School of Creative Leadership, 112
tiered huddles, 141
tools, crisis leadership, 17
training
    Federal Emergency Management Agency (FEMA), 166
    NIMs, 261
Trait Theory of Leadership, 106
transactional leadership style, 111
Transactional Theory of Leadership, 108
transdisciplinary concept, 180
Transformational Theory of Leadership, 108

transparency, 3, 32, 58
   communication, 221
   multifaceted communication, 153–154
trauma, 232–237
   coping, 236–237
   definition of, 232
   positive outcomes to, 240
   posttraumatic growth (PTG) theory, 234–235 (see also posttraumatic growth (PTG) theory)
   resilience, 233
triaging priorities, 6–7
trust
   collaboration and, 174–176
   mutual, 117–118, 122
trusting instinct, 70

U

University of Pennsylvania, 89
unknowns/knowns, 91, 92
Upholder (leadership), 269–270
US Department of Health and Human Services, 196
US Department of Transportation, 165
Useem, Michael, 89
US Food and Drug Administration, 207

V

vaccine mandates, 265. See also Covid-19 pandemic
values, shared commitments, 114–116, 122
valuing expertise, 117–118
visible power concept, 28
vision, shared commitments, 114–116, 122

W

Watson, Jean, 267
wave mindset, 262
   mental and physical resets, 262
   opportunity to change roles, 263–264
   reflection and re-evaluation, 263
Welch, Jack, 83
welcoming (mentorship), 38
Wharton School, 89
White House 2019 Novel Coronavirus Task Force, 207
World Health Organization (WHO), 83, 206, 207
Wuhan, China, 206. See also Covid-19 pandemic

X–Y–Z

Yoshino, Kenji, 35

Zoom, 63. See also communication

www.ingramcontent.com/pod-product-compliance
Lightning Source LLC
Chambersburg PA
CBHW071400300426
44114CB00016B/2124